Introductory Medical Statistics

Introductory
Medical Statistics

R. F. Mould

MSc, PhD, MInstP, AFIMA

Principal Physicist, Westminster Hospital
Hon. Lecturer in Medical Statistics,
Westminster Medical School, University of London

with a Foreword by

Professor Sir David Smithers
MD, FRCP, FRCS, FRCR

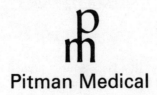

Pitman Medical

First Published 1976

Pitman Medical Publishing Co Ltd
42 Camden Road, Tunbridge Wells,
Kent TN1 2QD

Associated Companies

UNITED KINGDOM
Pitman Publishing Ltd, London
Focal Press Ltd, London

USA
Pitman Publishing Corporation, California
Fearon Publishers Inc, California

AUSTRALIA
Pitman Publishing Pty Ltd, Melbourne

CANADA
Pitman Publishing, Toronto
Copp Clark Publishing, Toronto

EAST AFRICA
Sir Isaac Pitman and Sons Ltd, Nairobi

SOUTH AFRICA
Pitman Publishing Co SA (Pty) Ltd, Johannesburg

NEW ZEALAND
Pitman Publishing NZ Ltd, Wellington

ISBN: 0 272 79397 3

Cat. No. 21 2445 81

Text set in 10/12 pt IBM Press Roman, printed by photolithography,
and bound in Great Britain at The Pitman Press, Bath

Contents

Foreword

We improve the efficiency of practice through the acquisition of information, whether this be thoughtfully accumulated or subconsciously absorbed. Experience is gained and impressions are formed which lead to changes in the conduct of our affairs. However, impressions have a tendency to confirm the notions we treasure and trial and error, the standard mode of progress, may prove costly in medicine in terms of suffering as well as in waste of time and resources. To get the best out of this system it has, therefore, to be refined and tested, with impartiality.

Statistics, which Lancelot Hogben called 'The Arithmetic of Human Welfare', add precision to the assessment of the significance of observations, the results of experiment and the meaning of relationships. They also aim to eliminate emotional pre-judgements, banish wishful thinking and allow results to be assessed with accuracy and checked by others. Laplace is quoted in Chapter 4 as saying that 'The theory of probability is only common sense reduced to calculation'. Perhaps we might suggest that statistics are observations elevated so as to make better sense.

The importance of statistical study was first recognised by those who wished to wager on games of chance, but medicine has steadily, if rather leisurely, exhibited a growing interest in the handling of matters of size and order so as to employ to better advantage the range of our experience, the extent of our information about the present and the feasibility of our ideas about the future. The introduction into medical examinations of questions about statistics has high-lighted the fact that, to be taken seriously as a reporter of work done and an advocate of change in medical practice today, demands a high standard both of scientific preparation and of presentation which will allow results to be checked and theories tested.

In this introduction to medical statistics, Richard Mould has written a book which is both timely and useful; such an account has long been needed and the task has been most skilfully performed. He has had the great advantage of working under Professor W. V. Mayneord and Professor J. W. Boag, two men renowned for their pioneer work in medical physics who directed their originality and their expertise so ably towards the practical applications of their work. Thus this book reflects an understanding of medical needs derived from day to day co-operation with doctors. The author also acquired an appreciation of the necessity for a solid foundation in basic principles learned from his earliest days in medical physics. With its clear text, 40 diagrams and classified index it will be of great value, not least to the less mathematically inclined of doctors who have in the past tended to shun a study they can no longer afford to neglect. I am delighted to have been asked to write a foreword to this admirable book by a former colleague. I wish it had been available to me when I was starting in medicine.

Professor Sir David Smithers
MD, FRCP, FRCS, FRCR

Preface

It is only relatively recently that medical statistics has featured to any great extent in MB, BS, MRCP and FRCR examinations; reflecting an increased awareness of the need to quantify clinical impressions accurately. To achieve this, a knowledge of various statistical tests and mathematical distributions is required, together with an understanding of the basic concepts of probability and statistical significance. Without a firm grasp of these concepts, formulae might be applied under inappropriate circumstances, leading to false conclusions. To avoid this situation I have included several introductory sections in the book, notably the majority of Chapter 6 which precedes discussion on the specific χ^2-, t- and F-tests. I have tried to take into account many doctors' aversion to mathematics and have kept calculations to a minimum, using simple numbers as a starting point wherever possible. However, in a book on statistics, some mathematics must be included!

Calculation schedules have been included for standard deviation (Tables 2.4 and 2.5); binomial probabilities (Table 5.3); χ^2-test (Table 7.1); contingency tables (Tables 7.7 to 7.9); paired and unpaired t-tests (Table 8.2); method of least squares (Table 9.2); and regression coefficient (Table 9.3). In this manner it is hoped that after understanding the background to the test, readers will be able to follow the necessary mathematical steps easily when using their own data.

Tables for the area under a normal curve, and for critical values of the χ^2, t and F statistics have intentionally been kept brief, since exhaustive tables are available in a booklet called Cambridge Elementary Statistical Tables (Lindley and Miller, 1968, *Cambridge University Press*).

The idea for this book arose out of a course of lectures given at Westminster in conjunction with Professor M. D. Milne, Professor of Medicine, to MB, BS students during 1974 and 1975. An elementary and inexpensive textbook was requested by the students but almost all were either too comprehensive and mathematical, or devoted to only one particular aspect of medicine.

The examples chosen to illustrate the first nine chapters have been taken from the general field of medicine, but those in Chapter 10 and 11 are mainly from oncology. This is intended to make them especially relevant for the FRCR examination, in which questions regularly appear on the design of clinical trials and calculation of survival times.

R. F. Mould, Westminster, January 1976

To
Timothy
Fiona
&
Jane

Acknowledgements

I would like to thank my colleagues at Westminster, in particular Dr J. P. Nicholson, Mrs T. M. Hearnden, Mr D. J. Brown and Dr M. Bakowski for many helpful discussions during the preparation of this book. I am grateful to the medical students, registrars and consultants who provided the initial audience and assisted with constructive criticisms.

I would also like to record my thanks to Professor J. W. Boag of the Royal Marsden Hospital: Institute of Cancer Research, who first stimulated my interest in medical statistics and provided me with my initial opportunity to work in the field.

I am also grateful to Miss V. S. Waters for her expertise in typing the manuscript, to Miss A. Corrigan who helped with the various stages of proof reading, and to Miss J. G. Mould of Akaroa, New Zealand for the genealogical data in Table 7.4. I am also very grateful to Mr D. Dickens, Mr S. Neal and Mr R. Addicott of Pitman Medical, for their help and consideration in the preparation of the final manuscript.

Tables 3.1, 7.2, 8.3 and 8.4 are based on data in Tables III, IV, III and V of Fisher and Yates: *Statistical Tables for Biological, Agricultural and Medical Research*, published by Longman Group Ltd., London, (previously published by Oliver and Boyd, Edinburgh), and by permission of the authors and publishers. I am grateful to the Literary Executor of the late Sir Ronald A. Fisher, FRS and to Dr. Frank Yates, FRS for their permission to reprint data from the 6th edition (1974) of their book.

Chapter 1

Data Presentation

When it is necessary to convey facts, theories or points of view to an audience, clarity of presentation is essential and this is never more true than in the field of statistics. None of the methods of display described in this chapter will be suitable for all situations, but there are sufficient to enable a choice to be made in most cases.

Pie Diagram

A pie diagram is a circle divided into segmental areas representing proportions. Since a circle consists of 360 degrees, the segments are calculated by dividing these 360° into the relevant proportions. For example, if there are to be three segments representing 10, 30 and 60 per cent proportions, they are calculated as follows: 10 per cent of 360° = 36°, 30 per cent of 360° = 108°, 60 per cent of 360° = 216°. Figure 1.1 is an example of a pie diagram.

Figure 1.1
Proportion of congenital malformations by site, England and Wales, 1970

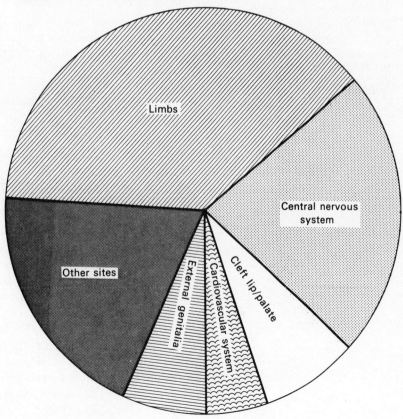

Dot Diagram

A dot diagram can be used to represent the state of a group of people at a given point in time, with different symbols describing different states. In Figure 1.2 the state of 20 patients up to three years after treatment is shown with the circles referring to those who are dead, and the triangles to those who are alive. The diagram is drawn using a yearly time scale. One advantage of this type of presentation is the large amount of information that can be clearly displayed and thus help with an overall assessment. Different colours can be used, as well as different shapes.

Figure 1.2
Dot diagram

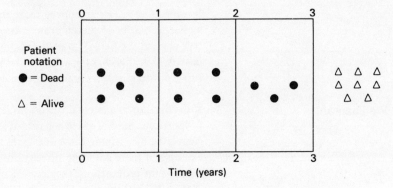

Patient notation

● = Dead

△ = Alive

Time (years)

Bar Chart

In a bar chart, the length of each bar represents the value of the variable of interest. In Figure 1.3, the variable is a hospital admission rate.

Figure 1.3
Bar chart of major causes of admission to hospital per 10 000 population in 1971, of the male age group 20–24, England and Wales

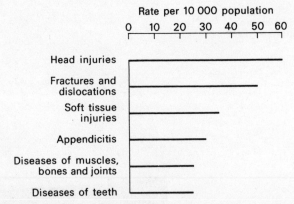

Rate per 10 000 population

Head injuries

Fractures and dislocations

Soft tissue injuries

Appendicitis

Diseases of muscles, bones and joints

Diseases of teeth

Frequency Table

Frequency is the term describing the occurrence of an event. If an event occurs 5 times out of every 10, then the frequency is 5 out of 10. (This is equivalent to 1 out of 2, or could be stated as a frequency of $\frac{1}{2}$ or 0.5.) Table 1.1 is a frequency table of recorded ages at diagnosis of stage 1 carcinoma cervix patients treated between 1945 and 1959 at London hospitals. The age range is given in the first column, and the frequency in the second column. The total frequency is the total number of patients, 580 in this example. To calculate the *cumulative frequency*, the frequencies of the second column are added consecutively. The cumulative frequency (C.F.) of 22 shows that '22 patients in the series had ages less than or equal to 29 years', the C.F. of 136 shows that '136 patients in the series had ages less than or equal to 39 years' . . . , etc. The *percentage cumulative frequency* in the fourth column is the cumulative frequency expressed as a percentage of the total (580) cases; e.g. (100 x 22/580) = 3.8%.

Table 1.1
Frequency table

Age Range (years)	Frequency	Cumulative Frequency	Percentage Cumulative Frequency
0—19	0	0	0
20—29	22	22	3.8%
30—39	114	136	23.4%
40—49	152	288	49.7%
50—59	150	438	75.5%
60—69	112	550	94.8%
70—79	29	579	99.8%
80—89	1	580	100 %
	Total = 580		

Histogram

In a histogram the height of each vertical block represents the value of the variable of interest in a similar manner to the length of a horizontal bar in a bar chart. Indeed, a bar chart can be thought of as a histogram turned on its side, with both vertical ends of each histogram block compressed together to form a single line. Figure 1.4 is an example of a histogram.

Figure 1.4
Histogram of age at menopause of 123 women with cancer of the uterine body (Data from Roberts D. W. T., *J. Obst. Gynaec. Brit. Comm.*, 1961, Vol. 68, p. 132)

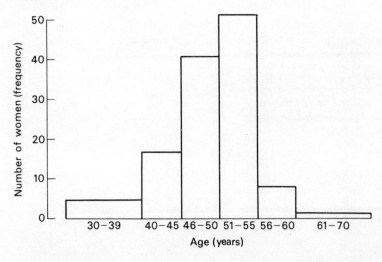

Frequency Polygon

If the mid-points of the tops of each histogram block are joined together by straight lines then the resultant pattern formed by the lines is called a frequency polygon.

Frequency Curve

The data in Table 1.1 are *observed* frequency data. It is possible, in some cases, to *fit* a *theoretical* curve to the observations which would then provide *expected* frequencies. Figure 1.5 shows such a curve superimposed on a histogram and is a *best fit* curve to the observations. It is similar to a *smoothed* frequency polygon. The frequency curve in Figure 1.5 is a special example called a *normal* curve and can be calculated using a particular mathematical formula (*see* Chapter 2).

Figure 1.5
Frequency curve and histogram
of age at diagnosis of stage 1
carcinoma cervix

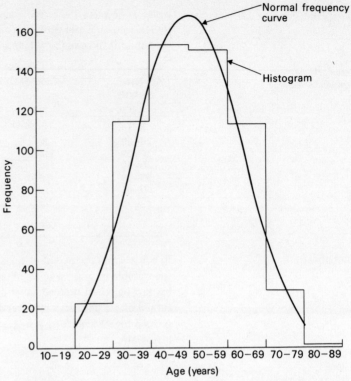

Figure 1.6
Mean height of boys between
birth and 12 years of age on
linear graph paper (Data
from Documenta Geigy

Scientific Tables, 7th edn,
1970, Courtesy Ciba-Geigy)

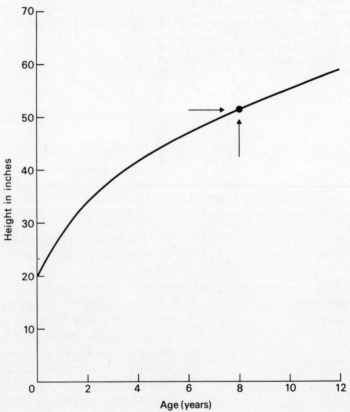

Graph Paper

LINEAR GRAPH PAPER Figure 1.6 is a graph showing the variation of height with age of boys from 0 to 12 years. The two arrows mark the height at age 8 years. A graph has two *axes*, in this example the vertical height axis, and the horizontal age axis. Each starts at 0, and this point 0 is called the *origin* of the graph. Convention describes the vertical axis as the *Y*-axis or *ordinate* axis, and the horizontal axis as the *X*-axis or the *abscissa* axis. Any point on the graph can be given co-ordinates, that is, can be specified by two values, which in Figure 1.6 are height and age. The *co-ordinates* of the arrowed point can be denoted in brackets: (8,51), with the *X*-value stated first and the *Y*-value stated second and separated from each other by a comma.

There are many types of graph paper and the simplest is *linear graph paper* such as in Figure 1.6. In this diagram, the distance on the age axis is the same for equal time intervals, i.e. for 0 to 2 years, 2 to 4 years and 4 to 6 years . . . , etc. The height axis also has a linear scale.

LOGARITHMIC GRAPH PAPER Figure 1.7 shows *log-linear graph*

Figure 1.7
Log-Linear graph paper

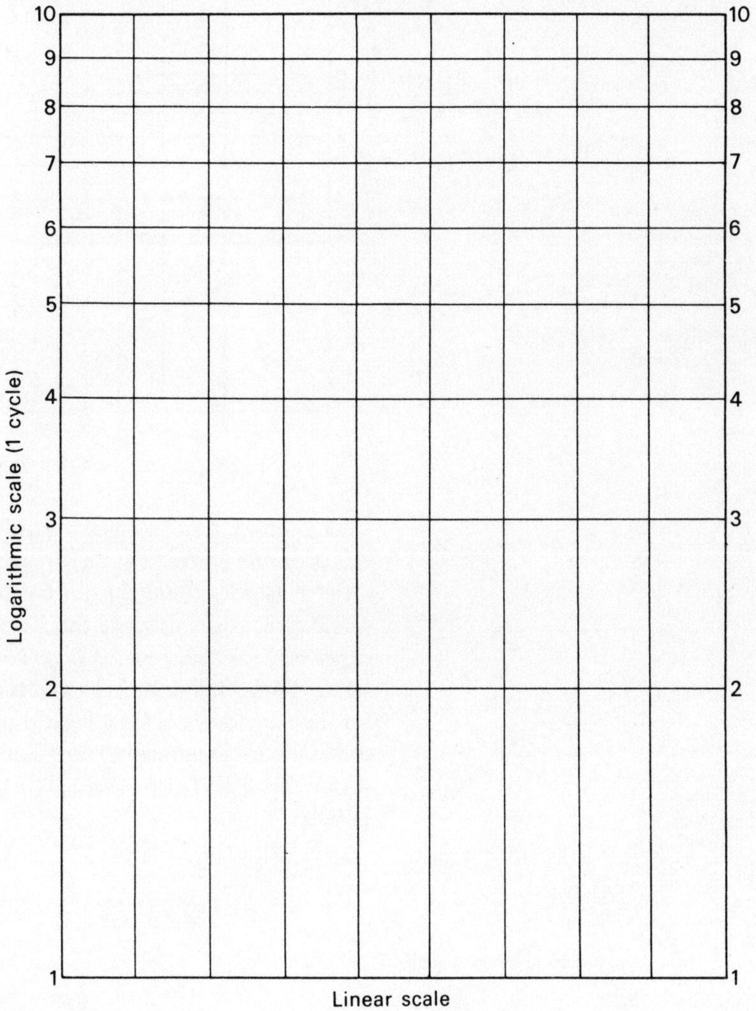

Logarithmic scale (1 cycle)

Linear scale

paper which has a *linear X*-scale and a *logarithmic Y*-scale. For the vertical logarithmic axis, equal *Y*-intervals, i.e. from 1 to 2, 2 to 3, 3 to 4, 4 to 5, ... etc do *not* correspond to equal distances on the *Y*-axis as they do for a linear scale. Figure 1.8 shows *log-log graph paper* with a logarithmic scale on both axes. The term *cycles* refers to the number of sets of 1 to 10 on an axis, and Figure 1.8 would therefore be classified *log 2 cycles by log 2 cycles*.

Figure 1.8
Log-Log graph paper

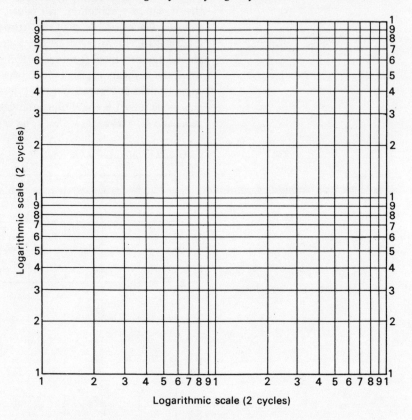

One advantage of using a logarithmic scale is that a wider range of values can be plotted than when using linear graph paper. For example, if the *Y*-values extended from say 20 to 1 000, linear graph paper would either have to make the *Y*-scale very compressed or the graph paper very tall, whereas *log 2 cycles* in Figure 1.8 could extend from 10 to 100 for the first cycle, and then through 200, 300, ... to 1 000 for the second cycle. On a logarithmic scale, the values assigned to successive cycle numbers 1 to 10, increase by powers of 10, for example, within the series 0.1 to 1.0; 1.0 to 10; 10 to 100; 100 to 1 000; 1 000 to 10 000.

Chapter 2

Describing Curves

To describe a curve so that it can be reproduced, a quantitative description is needed. The terms *curve* and *distribution* used here are synonymous, in the sense that a particular curve depicts the distribution of a quantity such as age in Figure 1.5, and the diagram is called a *distribution curve*.

A curve is drawn relative to two axes, *X* and *Y*, and the description of the curve must include information about both its *position* and its *shape*.

Curve Position: The Mean, Mode and Median

There are three important commonly used measures of position: the arithmetic mean, mode and median. For the data in Table 2.1 the *arithmetic mean* or *average* duration of symptoms is the sum of all the durations divided by the total number of patients; i.e.

$$\frac{(7 + 6 + 3 + 11 + 5 + 7 + 7 + 9 + 6 + 5)}{10} = \frac{66}{10} = 6.6 \ weeks$$

The *mode* of the distribution is the observation that occurs most frequently. This is *7 weeks*, which occurs three times. The *median* is the middle valued observation when all the observations are *ranked* in

Table 2.1
Observations

Duration of symptoms prior to treatment (Data for 10 patients)
7 6 3 11 5 7 7 9 6 5   weeks

order of value. If the total number of observations is even — as in Table 2.1 — the median is the value between the two middle observations. In the example, the *median* is 'between 6 and 7 weeks', Table 2.2.

Table 2.2
Ranked observations

Duration of symptoms prior to treatment, arranged in ranking order
3 5 5 6 6 7 7 7 9 11   weeks
↑
MEDIAN

For the special case when the frequency curve is *symmetrical*,

THE MEAN = THE MODE = THE MEDIAN

Formula 2.1
Mean, mode and median

However, most distributions are at least slightly asymmetrical, in which case, the formula should be used:

Formula 2.2
Mean, mode and median

$$\text{MEAN} - \text{MODE} = 3 \times (\text{MEAN} - \text{MEDIAN})$$

In the example, the mean was 6.6 and the mode was 7. Thus, using Formula 2.2 $[6.6 - 7] = 3 \times [6.6 - \text{median}]$ and the median equals 6.7 weeks, which agrees with the earlier statement 'between 6 and 7'.

Curve Shape: Skewness, Variance and Standard Deviation

In the preceding example it was shown that: mode = 7 weeks, median = 6.7 weeks, mean = 6.6 weeks, and thus:

[Mode] is greater than [Median] is greater than [Mean].

The distribution of symptom durations is therefore *pushed over towards the right* as in the lowest curve of Figure 2.1. The terminology for asymmetry in a distribution curve is *skewness*. When the *mode* or peak of the curve is pushed to the right, the distribution is called *negatively skewed* and when pushed to the left is called *positively skewed*. A *symmetrical* curve has no skewness.

Figure 2.1
Curve shapes

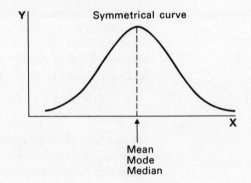

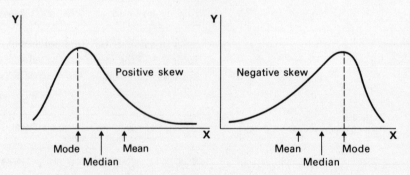

Symmetry or asymmetry will not completely describe the shape of a curve since the mode could be either very pointed or very flat. This *peak property* of the curve is called *kurtosis*.

When discussing the relationship between the mean, mode and median, skewness and kurtosis have been described. However, the most important and most useful parameter of curve shape is *standard deviation*.

To explain this term, consider four patients with varying symptom durations prior to treatment, Table 2.3.

Table 2.3
Data

Duration of symptoms prior to treatment, (Data for 4 patients, $N = 4$)
4 5 6 9 weeks

The *arithmetic mean* for the data in Table 2.3 is 6 weeks. Call this $\bar{x}$ and the individual durations x, that is, $x_1 = 4$ weeks ... $x_4 = 9$ weeks, where the jth duration is x_j, using the same terminology. The *deviation* of x_j, *from the mean* duration, $\bar{x}$, is $(x_j - \bar{x})$. If this quantity, the *deviation from the mean*, is squared, $(x_j - \bar{x})^2$, and summed for all the $N = 4$ x-values, the sum total of all the $(x_j - \bar{x})^2$ values divided by $(N - 1)$ is called the *variance*. The *square root of the variance* is called the *standard deviation*. Figure 2.2 shows this procedure in block diagram format.

Figure 2.2
Calculation of standard deviation

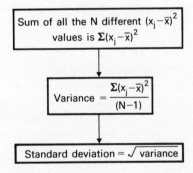

The boxes read:

Sum of all the N different $(x_j - \bar{x})^2$ values is $\Sigma(x_j - \bar{x})^2$

$$\text{Variance} = \frac{\Sigma(x_j - \bar{x})^2}{(N-1)}$$

$$\text{Standard deviation} = \sqrt{\text{variance}}$$

There are two methods of working out the arithmetic required for finding the *standard deviation*. The first is to use directly the formula in Figure 2.2 where the sign Σ means *the sum of all the* .... This direct method is shown in Table 2.4.

Formula 2.3
Standard deviation

$$\text{Standard Deviation} = \sqrt{\frac{\Sigma(x_j - \bar{x})^2}{(N-1)}}$$

The second method designed for a quicker calculation, gives the standard deviation in the form:

Formula 2.4
Standard deviation

$$\text{Standard Deviation} = \sqrt{\frac{\Sigma(x^2) - \frac{(\Sigma x)^2}{N}}{(N-1)}}$$

and is shown in Table 2.5. In Formula 2.4, the mean, $\bar{x}$, is not mentioned explicitly, but the formula is, nevertheless, only Formula 2.3 with the algebra rearranged.

Table 2.4
Calculation of standard deviation using Formula 2.3

Symptom Duration (x_j)	$(x_j - \bar{x})$	$(x_j - \bar{x})^2$	
4	−2	4	
5	−1	1	
6	0	0	
9	+3	9	Standard deviation =
$\Sigma(x) = 24$		$\Sigma(x_j - \bar{x})^2$	$\sqrt{\dfrac{14}{(4-1)}} = 2.2$
$x = (24/4)$			
$= 6$		$= 14$	

Table 2.5
Calculation of standard deviation using Formula 2.4

Symptom Duration (x_j)	$(x_j)^2$	
4	16	
5	25	
6	36	
9	81	Standard deviation = $\sqrt{\dfrac{158 - \dfrac{(24)^2}{4}}{(4-1)}} = 2.2$
$\Sigma(x) = 24$	$\Sigma(x^2)$	
$\bar{x} = (24/4)$	$= 158$	
$= 6$		

Chapter 3

Normal and Lognormal Curves

Introduction

When a frequency curve is described as normal, the term is *not* used in the sense that it is the distribution curve which is found to represent more observational data than any other type of distribution curve — but rather in the sense that it is a special type of symmetrical curve. In fact, the *lognormal* distribution curve could be considered to represent more data patterns of observations than the *normal*. Examples of frequency distributions which may sometimes be approximated by a normal curve are those of (*a*) height, (*b*) blood pressure and (*c*) mean red blood cell volume in a population of normal people. Examples of frequency distributions that may sometimes be approximated by lognormal curves, are (*a*) relation between time and death rate of bacteria, (*b*) survival time subsequent to treatment of certain groups of cancer patients who die with cancer present, and (*c*) distribution of sensitivities to drugs among individual animals of the same species, as measured by the dose required to cause some definite effect.

Mathematical Formulae

THE NORMAL DISTRIBUTION   Any well-defined distribution such as the *normal* also called the Gaussian distribution, will always have an associated mathematical formula to enable its shape to be calculated and then drawn graphically. Formula 3.1 is the simplest formula for a normal curve.

$$Y = \frac{1}{\sqrt{2\pi}} \cdot e^{-\frac{1}{2}X^2}$$

Formula 3.1
The normal curve
$\mu = 0$, $\sigma = 1$

e is an *exponential* and $e^{-\frac{1}{2}X^2}$ is called e to the $[-\frac{1}{2}X^2]$, $e^0 = 1$, $e^{-\infty} = 0$, where ∞ is the symbol for infinity, $e^{+\infty} = \infty$, $e^1 = e = 2.7183$. π is a constant equal to 3.1416.

For the normal curve of Formula 3.1, (*a*) the *mean*, *mode* and *median* values of Y occur when X = 0; and (*b*) the *standard deviation* (denoted in future by the Greek letter σ) equals 1. The general mathematical formula for the *normal* curve is given in Formula 3.2, where the *standard deviation* is denoted by σ and the mean by the Greek letter μ. In the general curve, the *mean* is located on the X-axis at $X = \mu$.

$$Y = \frac{1}{\sigma\sqrt{2\pi}} \cdot e^{-\frac{1}{2}\frac{(X-\mu)^2}{\sigma^2}}$$

Formula 3.2
The normal curve

If we say that $\mu = 0$, then Formula 3.2 becomes:

$$Y = \frac{1}{\sigma\sqrt{2\pi}} \cdot e^{-\frac{1}{2}\frac{X^2}{\sigma^2}}$$

Formula 3.3
The normal curve

Standard deviation is a measure of curve spread, and any alterations in σ will consequently alter the spread of the curve. Figure 3.1 shows a series of normal curves with different σ-values.

Figure 3.1
Normal curves with constant
mean μ, and variable standard
deviation σ

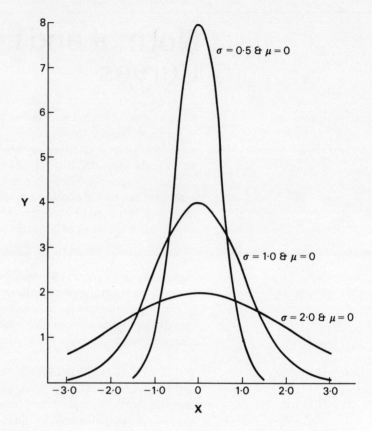

THE LOGNORMAL DISTRIBUTION   The formula for the general lognormal distribution with *mean M* and *standard deviation S* is Formula 3.4.

Formula 3.4
The lognormal curve

$$Y = \frac{1}{S\sqrt{2\pi}} \cdot \frac{1}{T} \cdot e^{-\frac{1}{2}\frac{[(\log_e T) - M]^2}{S^2}}$$

Figure 3.2 shows a series of lognormal curves with the same *standard deviation S*, but different values of the *mean, M*. As *M* decreases, the *mode* of the curve moves towards the left and the peak of the curve becomes sharper. For the *normal* curve, (mean) = (mode) and hence the mean value of *X* always corresponds to the peak of the distribution. The *lognormal* distribution, however, is a skewed distribution, where the mean is *not* the same as the mode. For a constant value of the mean *M*, and variable standard deviation *S*, the position of the mode with respect to the *X*-axis, does *not* remain the same, Figure 3.3, as it did for the normal curves in Figure 3.1.

Figure 3.2
Lognormal curves with
constant standard deviation,
S, and variable mean, *M*

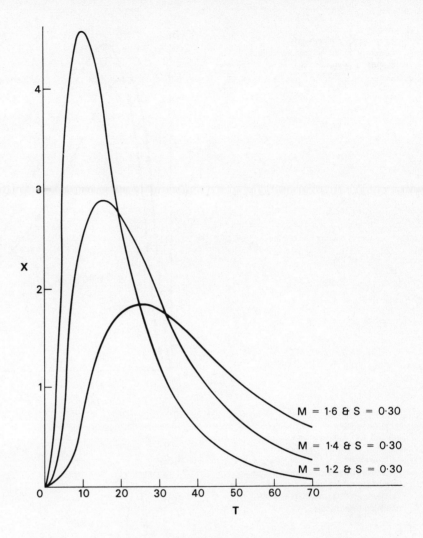

X

T

M = 1·6 & S = 0·30

M = 1·4 & S = 0·30

M = 1·2 & S = 0·30

Logarithmic Transformation of a Linear Scale

The word *transformation* is statistical terminology, for *change*. In Figure 1.7 a *linear* scale was shown for the graph paper *X*-axis, and a *logarithmic* scale for the graph paper *Y*-axis. In Figure 1.8 the *Y*-axis was still logarithmic but the *X*-axis had been changed from linear to logarithmic.

Figure 3.4 is a histogram of survival times of patients treated for cancer who died with their cancer present — *see* lognormal example (*b*) on page 11. This histogram is drawn on a *linear scale* with survival time (*X*-axis) intervals between 0 and 16 years. The histogram is redrawn in Figure 3.5, on a *logarithmic scale*, in this case using *logarithms to base 1.5.* The first interval is 6 to 9, since $(1.5 \times 6) = 9$; the second interval is 9 to $13\frac{1}{2}$, since $(1.5 \times 9) = 13\frac{1}{2}, \ldots$ etc.

In Figure 3.5 it is seen that the smooth curve superimposed on the histogram is the bell-shaped normal curve, although in this example it is the *lognormal* curve, since the survival time axis is a *logarithmic* and *not* a linear scale.

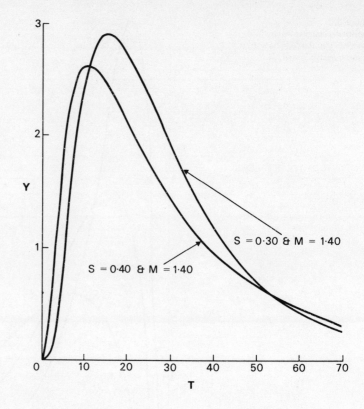

Figure 3.3
Lognormal curves with
constant mean M, and variable
standard deviation, S

S = 0·30 & M = 1·40

S = 0·40 & M = 1·40

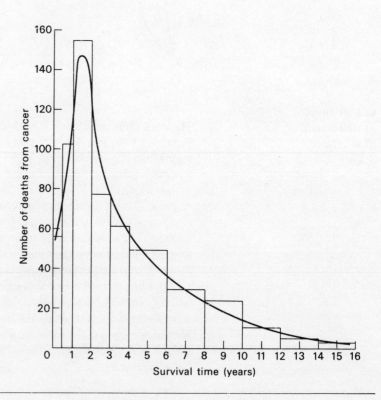

Figure 3.4
Survival time distribution of
583 stage 2 carcinoma cervix
patients, with time axis drawn
using a linear scale

Figure 3.5
Survival time distribution of
583 stage 2 carcinoma cervix
patients, with time axis drawn
using a logarithmic scale

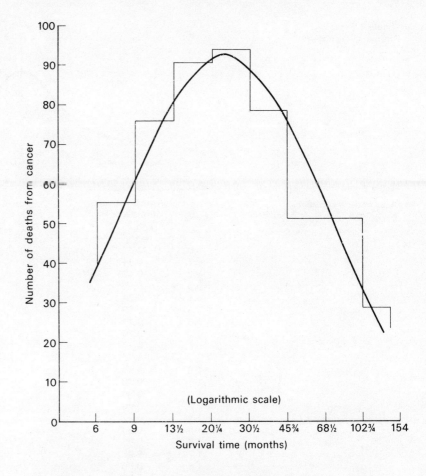

The Area Underneath a Normal (or Lognormal) Curve

In Chapter 4 we shall be dealing with *probability* and shall be using the *normal* distribution as a probability distribution, and we will need to calculate areas beneath the curve.

The mathematical symbol for the statement *the area under curve Y between the limits X = a and X = b* is

$$\int_{X=a}^{X=b} Y \cdot dx$$

where $\int$ is known as an integral sign. In *probability* we shall learn that the *total* probability is considered always equal to 1, and hence for a probability distribution, the total area under the curve, the integral from minus infinity to plus infinity, is always equal to 1.

The area beneath the normal curve of Formula 3.1 we will denote by the letter *P*, Formula 3.5 and by the shaded area in Figure 3.6. This is also given in Table 3.1. The unshaded area in Figure 3.6 will equal $(1 - P)$.

Formula 3.5
Area under the normal curve with $\mu = 0$, $\sigma = 1$

$$P = \int_{X=-\infty}^{X=\zeta} \frac{1}{\sqrt{2\pi}} \cdot e^{-\frac{1}{2}X^2} \cdot dx$$

15

Figure 3.6
Normal curve notation

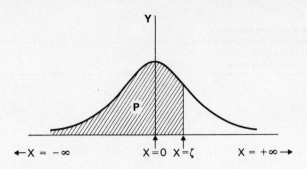

Table 3.1

Area under a normal
curve

ζ	Area P between limits $X = -\infty$ and $X = \zeta$
0.0	0.50
0.1	0.54
0.2	0.58
0.3	0.62
0.4	0.66
0.5	0.69
0.6	0.73
0.7	0.76
0.8	0.79
0.9	0.82
1.0	0.84
1.1	0.86
1.2	0.88
1.3	0.90
1.4	0.92
1.5	0.93
1.6	0.95
1.7	0.96
1.8	0.96
1.9	0.97
2.0	0.98
2.5	0.99
3.0	0.999

It is also noted that for the normal curve, there is an easily understood meaning for *standard deviation*, Table 3.2 and Figure 3.7.

Table 3.2
An explanation of
standard deviation

Standard Deviation Limits		Area beneath the normal curve between the S.D. limits
$+1\sigma$	& -1σ	68%
$+1.645\sigma$	& -1.645σ	90%
$+1.96\sigma$	& -1.96σ	95%
$+2\sigma$	& -2σ	$95\frac{1}{2}\%$
$+3\sigma$	& -3σ	$99\frac{3}{4}\%$

Probability Graph Paper

Linear and logarithmic graph paper have already been described, but there is also an additional type of paper called *probability graph paper*. For the *normal* distribution, this provides a simple graphical method

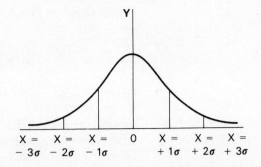

Figure 3.7
The normal curve with the
X-axis in units of standard
deviation, σ

of estimating the parameters μ and σ of Formula 3.2 — if the distribution *is* normal — and for the *lognormal* distribution, it provides a simple method of estimating M and S — if the distribution *is* lognormal. The graph paper has the same probability X-axis scale for both normal *and* lognormal, but different Y-axes — linear for the normal (*arithmetic probability paper*) and logarithmic for the lognormal (*logarithmic probability paper*).

Figure 3.8 illustrates the use of arithmetic probability paper for the data of Table 1.1 where the parameter observed is age.

Figure 3.8
Graphical demonstration of
normality

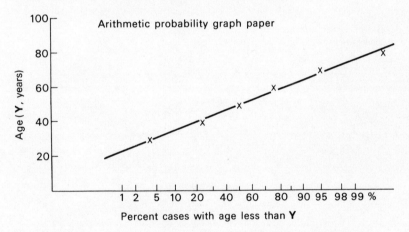

The mean, μ, of the normal distribution in Figure 3.8 will be that age which corresponds to the 50 per cent cumulative percentage value, since [mean = median] for the symmetrical normal distribution; μ is 49 years for this example. From Table 3.2 it is seen that 10 per cent of the observations lie at a distance from the mean which is greater than 1.645σ, and that half of these (5 per cent) are smaller than μ and half (5 per cent) are larger than μ. The *standard deviation*, σ, may therefore be calculated using Formula 3.6.

$$[1.645] = \left\{ \begin{matrix} Y\text{-value corresponding} \\ \text{to 95\% cumulation} \end{matrix} - \begin{matrix} Y\text{-value corresponding} \\ \text{to 50\% cumulation} \end{matrix} \right\}$$

Formula 3.6
Standard deviation
(normal curve)

$$\sigma = \frac{(Y_{95\%} - \mu)}{1.645}$$

17

For the sample in Figure 3.8, Y = age and $Y_{95\%}$ = 68 years and μ = 49 years, therefore:

$$\sigma = \frac{(68 - 49)}{1.645} = 11.6$$

Figure 3.9 illustrates the use of logarithmic probability paper and uses the data of Figure 3.4 to calculate a percentage cumulative frequency in a similar manner to Table 1.1. The mean, M, of the lognormal distribution corresponds to the 50 per cent cumulative percentage value (M = 23 months), and the standard deviation, S, is calculated in a similar manner to the preceding example, using Formula 3.7, and remembering to use $Y_{95\%}$ and $M(= Y_{50\%})$ as logarithms to base 10.

Formula 3.7
Standard deviation
(logarithmic curve)

M = 23 months, $Y_{95\%}$ = 160 months

$$S = \frac{[\log_{10}(Y_{95\%}) - \log_{10}(M)]}{1.645}$$

$$S = \frac{(2.2041 - 1.3617)}{1.645} = 0.51$$

Figure 3.9
Graphical demonstration of
log-normality

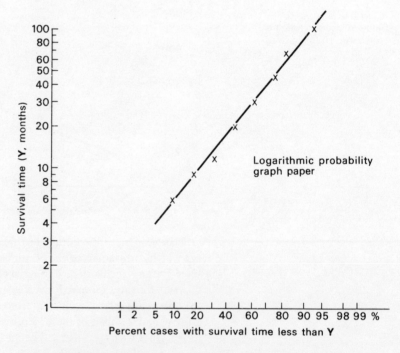

The two examples chosen did approximate to straight lines on the probability graph paper, Figure 3.8 and Figure 3.9. If, however, we had tested the Figure 3.9 data which is *lognormal* on *normal arithmetic* probability graph paper, then a curve would have been obtained, Figure 3.10. The line is distinctly *concave* — indicating that the data is *positively skewed* and not normal. If the curve had been *convex*, the data would have been *negatively skewed*.

Figure 3.10
Graphical plot of skewed,
non-normal data

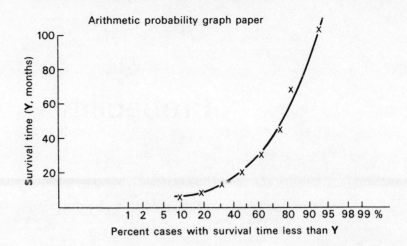

Arithmetic probability graph paper

Chapter 4

Probability

The theory of probability is only common sense reduced to calculation, it exhibits with accuracy what reasonable minds feel by a kind of instinct, without being able to describe it to themselves.

Laplace, French Mathematician, 1749–1827

Introduction to Probability

Vague probability statements based on personal assessment of situations are often heard, such as 'it is *likely* to rain tomorrow', 'there is a good *chance* of the price of food rising still further', 'football team A will *probably* beat team B', '. . . leave it to *chance*'. There are also everyday sayings which are supposed to link the *probability* of a future event with a current observation; that is, a statement of *conditional probability*. An example is 'red sky at night, shepherds' delight', implying good weather the following day. Such statements are *imprecise*, and *mathematical* probability attempts to enumerate the *chances for and against* and thus present a more *precise* and quantitative view.

The Two Laws of Mathematical Probability

Events occur either *simultaneously* or *consecutively*, and if we need to calculate a *total probability* to describe in numbers the likelihood of a series of events occurring, then the method of calculation (addition or multiplication) will depend upon how the events occur, that is, whether *simultaneously* or *consecutively*.

The two fundamental laws are given in Table 4.1, where the word *independent* is used with its ordinary English meaning.

Table 4.1

Laws of mathematical probability

LAW 1	*EXAMPLE*
The probability of occurrence of one or other of a number of *independent* events, only one of which can occur at a time, is the sum of probabilities of the separate events.	When throwing a die, each number 1 to 6 has an equally likely chance of turning up. A 5 and a 6 cannot both turn up in a single throw. However, the probability of *either* a 5 *or* a 6 turning up is $$\frac{1}{6} + \frac{1}{6} = \frac{1}{3}$$
LAW 2	*EXAMPLE*
The probability of the *simultaneous* occurrence of a number of *independent* events is the product of their separate probabilities.	When throwing two dice, there are 36 equally likely possibilities, Figure 4.1, and of these, only one is favourable to a double six. The probability of a double six is $$\frac{1}{6} \times \frac{1}{6} = \frac{1}{36}$$

Figure 4.1
An example of law 2 of
mathematical probability

With a simultaneous throw of two dice
the probability of a
double six

 is

1 chance in 36 attempts

A die has six sides, and thus the *chance* or *probability* of any of the sides falling face up in a single throw is *one in six* (1/6).

The expression *mutually exclusive* is a term related to events such that if one event happens, it is impossible for the second event to occur. In terms of a *single* die throw, throwing a 6 and throwing a 5 are mutually exclusive events since the experiment consisted of a *single* throw with only one die.

Examples in Probability

In statistics, probability can be thought of as *proportionate frequency,* referred to an infinite population. Taking as an example, a horse race in which the probability of *XYZ* winning is 1/5; we can imagine a very large number of horse races, all run under the same conditions. This is the *infinite population*, and in 1/5th of these races, horse *XYZ* wins. The more identical races run, the closer the proportion of races won by horse *XYZ* will be to 1/5th. Another example would be the probability of surviving a particular operation. An estimate of the survival probability could be obtained from a sample of three patients, but a more accurate value would be obtained with a larger sample of say 100 patients.

> Probability = 0 means that the event *never* occurs
> Probability = 1 means that the event *always* occurs

In other words, probability is expressed numerically on a scale from 0 to 1. When a normal distribution is to be used as a probability distribution, with the area under the curve representing numerical probability values, the total area will be 1. When the total area under a curve is equal to 1, the curve is said to be *normalised*. The information in Table 3.2 is re-stated in Table 4.2 using probability terminology for an event known to follow a normal probability distribution pattern.

Table 4.2
Probability and area
under the normal curve

The probability of an event occurring within
the range
$[\pm n \cdot \sigma]$
is equal to the area under the normal curve
between the limits
$[\pm n \cdot \sigma]$

$n \cdot \sigma$	Probability
1σ	0.68
1.645σ	0.90
1.96σ	0.95
2σ	0.96
3σ	1.00

Suppose that the heights of a group of men can be represented by a normal distribution with a mean of 183 cm (6 feet) and standard deviation, σ, of 7 cm. From the information in Table 4.2 we can make the following probability statements:

(a) 68 per cent of the group will have a height in the range 183 cm ± 7 cm.

(b) Only 10 per cent of the group will have heights either greater than 183 cm + $11\frac{1}{2}$ cm, or less than 183 cm − $11\frac{1}{2}$ cm (7 x 1.645 = $11\frac{1}{2}$).

(c) Virtually all members of the group will have heights within the range 183 cm ± 21 cm.

To illustrate the two laws in Table 4.1, suppose that we are interested in the successful outcome of a hypothetical operation, which depends upon several factors including age of the patient, sex, and whether the operation has been attempted previously with unsuccessful results. For this example the numerical values will be attached to the various separate probabilities.

Table 4.3
Data for a probability calculation

Factor	Probability of success
Age less than 50	4 out of 5
Age greater than 50	2 out of 5
Male	4 out of 5
Female	3 out of 5
No previous operation	3 out of 4
Previous operation	1 out of 2

The probability of success for a male, under 50, first operation, will be calculated using Law 2 since all the three factors can occur simultaneously. Thus:

$$\text{Pr[Success]}_{\substack{\text{Under 50, male} \\ \text{First operation}}} = \left(\frac{4}{5} \times \frac{4}{5} \times \frac{3}{4}\right) = \frac{12}{25}$$

Similarly, using Law 2,

$$\text{Pr[Success]}_{\substack{\text{Over 50, male} \\ \text{Second operation}}} = \left(\frac{2}{5} \times \frac{4}{5} \times \frac{1}{2}\right) = \frac{4}{25}$$

Now suppose that we are considering both the previously mentioned males, and we wish to calculate the probability of a successful outcome of the operation in *either* one *or* the other of the patients. Law 1 is now required in which the individual probabilities of success are added:

$$\text{Pr[Success]}_{\substack{\text{Under 50, male, First operation} \\ or \\ \text{Over 50, male, second operation}}} = \frac{12}{25} + \frac{4}{25} = \frac{16}{25}$$

Chapter 5

The Binomial Distribution

**Permutations
and
Combinations**

A knowledge of *permutations* and *combinations* is necessary before the binomial distribution is discussed, since they are needed for the calculations involved with binomial problems. The difference between the two terms is that for *combinations* the order of objects *is not* important, whereas for *permutations* the order *is* important.

To illustrate this, consider three objects A, B and C. The group of three will be called a *set*, and a *permutation* is an arrangement of a set or part of a set. Thus, permutations of *two from three* are:

$$\boxed{AB \quad BA \quad AC \quad CA \quad BC \quad CB}$$ which are written $^3P_2$

That is, $^3P_2 = 6$

If we now consider a set of four objects A, B, C and D, then permutations of *three from four*, are:

$$\boxed{\begin{array}{cccccc} ABC & ACB & BAC & BCA & CAB & CBA \\ ABD & ADB & BAD & BDA & DAB & DBA \\ ACD & ADC & CAD & CDA & DAC & DCA \\ BCD & BDC & CBD & CDB & DBC & DCB \end{array}}$$ which are written $^4P_3$

A general formula for obtaining *r from n* permutations is:

**Formula 5.1
Permutations**

$$^nP_r = \frac{n!}{(n-r)!}$$

where $n!$ is called *n factorial* and $(1!) = 1$; $(2!) = 1 \times 2 = 2$; $(3!) = 1 \times 2 \times 3 = 6$; $(4!) = 1 \times 2 \times 3 \times 4 = 24$; $(n!) = (1 \times 2 \times 3 \times 4 \times 5 \times \ldots \times n)$. Formula 5.1 can be used for $^3P_2$ where $n = 3$ and $r = 2$,

$$^3P_2 = \frac{3!}{(3-2)!} = 6. \text{ For } ^4P_3 \text{ where } n = 4 \text{ and } r = 3, {}^4P_3 = \frac{4!}{(4-3)!} = 24.$$

The answers 6 and 24 can be checked by counting the permutations in the boxes.

For *combinations*, the order is *not* important, and thus in our first example, although *AB* and *BA* count as *two* permutations, they only count as *one* combination; similarly in the second example, *ABC*, *BCA* and *CAB* count as *three* permutations, but only as *one* combination. Thus, the combinations of *three from four* are:

$$\begin{array}{l} ABC \\ ABD \\ ACD \\ BCD \end{array}$$ which are written $^4C_3 = 4$

The general formula for obtaining *r from n* combinations is:

Formula 5.2
Combinations
(binomial coefficient)

$$^nC_r = \frac{n!}{r!\,(n-r)!}$$

There is an extra term ($r!$) in the denominator of Formula 5.2 compared with Formula 5.1, since there are always fewer combinations than permutations for the same *r from n*. An alternative symbolism for ^nC_r is $\begin{pmatrix} n \\ r \end{pmatrix}$.

In practice, the formulae are useful, since it is often too laborious to tabulate all the possible combinations or permutations.

For example, the number of ways in which two cards can be dealt from a pack of 52, when order does not matter, is $^{52}C_2$ or, using Formula 5.2 $\frac{52!}{(2! \times 50!)}$. Many terms will cancel out from numerator and denominator, leaving

$$^{52}C_2 = \frac{(52 \times 51)}{(2 \times 1)} = 1\,326$$

If we are interested in drawing the ace of hearts and king of hearts, either ace first *or* king first, then we have one chance of success in 1 326 tries. A more complicated example is the chance of a pontoon (an ace and a face card) and this is calculated as follows. There are twelve face cards and four aces in the pack, thus there are 48 different combinations which give a pontoon. The chance of drawing a pontoon is, therefore, 48 in 1 326, i.e. 48/1326, or *one in 27.6*, or *a probability of 0.036* or a probability of 3.6 per cent. *N.B.* This is the chance of the first *two* cards to be dealt being a pontoon.

The Binomial Distribution

The *binomial distribution* refers to simple yes or no, black or white, 0 or 1, dead or alive situations where there are only *two* alternatives, and it can be used to determine whether the results observed in a *trial-experiment* situation could have occurred *randomly*. This is important because if the results could quite easily have occurred by chance, *no conclusions can be drawn*.

Suppose that we have a *trial* in which the *outcome* can only be one of two events, A or B, and let the *probability* of event A be (p). Since the *total probability = 1*, the probability of event B is $(1-p)$, and could be denoted (q). We could for example say that event A was success and event B failure, and so the binomial probability for success = p and the binomial probability of failure = q, where $p + q = 1$. Now suppose that the identical trial is conducted *n times*. This can be referred to as a *sample* of *n* trials. The problem which can be solved by *binomial* theory is:

> *What is the probability distribution of the numbers of successes (As) in the sample of n trials?*

If the number of As (successes) is equal to r, then the number of Bs (failures) will be equal to $(n - r)$. The *binomial distribution* gives the probability that the sample of n contains (r) As and $(n - r)$ Bs.

The binomial distribution can be written as Formula 5.3 where the first term ^nC_r can be recognised as a *combination* given by Formula 5.2.

Formula 5.3
Binomial
probability

$$\begin{array}{l}\text{Binomial}\\\text{Probability}\\\text{of } r \text{ successes}\\\text{in } n \text{ trials}\end{array} = {}^nC_r \cdot p^r \cdot (1 - p)^{n-r}$$

This *combination*, ^nC_r or $\binom{n}{r}$ is called the *binomial coefficient*, and it can be obtained using a diagram called *Pascal's triangle*, Fig. 5.1, without having to use Formula 5.2. In the triangle, the numbers can be extended *downwards*. Each entry is obtained as the sum of the two adjacent numbers of the line above. Thus, in the row for $n = 2$, the middle number 2 in the row 1 2 1 is obtained by $(1 + 1)$ from row $n = 1$. Similarly, the 5 in the row for $n = 5$ is obtained by $(1 + 4)$ from row $n = 4$. Each row contains the binomial coefficients ^nC_r for that particular value of n. Thus, for the row $n = 3$, there are four entries 1 3 3 1 which correspond to $^3C_0, ^3C_1, ^3C_2, ^3C_3$.

Before any examples of the use of the binomial are given, Table 5.1 summarises the three conditions under which a *trial* can be considered to be a *binomial* situation.

Table 5.1
Conditions for a
binomial trial

---
1. *The experiment consists of a fixed number of trials, n.*
---
2. *Each trial has only two possible outcomes, usually called success and failure.*
---
3. *The outcome of any trial is independent of the outcome of any other trial.*

Condition 3 in Table 5.1 for a trial with a pack of cards where *success* was signified by drawing an ace, would be satisfied, if after each draw the card chosen was replaced in the deck of cards before the next draw. Otherwise, the trials would *not* be independent, since the second trial would be related to the first because of the removal of the first card. If on the first draw the card was an ace, the initial probability of success, p, would be 4/52 and if there was no replacement, the probability of an ace for a second draw would be $p = 3/51$. This would not be a trial when the binomial distribution could be used since p must be the same throughout all the n binomial trials.

To illustrate the use of Formula 5.3 and Pascal's triangle, Figure 5.1, consider a simple experiment, Table 5.2. The data necessary for Formula 5.3 and Figure 5.1 is given in this table.

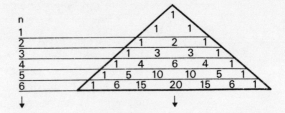

From Pascal's triangle for $n = 3$, the binomial coefficients ^nC_r are 1, 3, 3 and 1 for $r = 0, 1, 2$ and 3. The method of solution and answers to the problem are given in Table 5.3 and Figure 5.2.

Table 5.2
Description of a
binomial problem

Experiment	5 balls in an opaque box, 3 are red and 2 are black. Three balls are drawn successively, and after each has been drawn and recorded, it is replaced prior to the next draw.
Problem?	What is the probability that 0, 1, 2 or 3 red balls will be drawn.
Number of trials, n	$n = 3$
Probability of success, p	Pr (of a red outcome) $= p = 3/5$ Thus $(1 - p) = 2/5$

Table 5.3
Calculation of
binomial
probabilities

Value of r, the number of successes	^nC_r	p^r where $p = 3/5$	$(1 - p)^{n-r}$ where $n = 3$	Binomial probability from Formula 5.3
0	1	*1	8/125	8/125 = 0.06
1	3	3/5	4/25	36/125 = 0.29
2	3	9/25	2/5	54/125 = 0.43
3	1	27/125	*1	27/125 = 0.22

*Note $p^0 = (1 - p)^0 = 1$

A binomial situation of historical importance is the work of Jenner on smallpox vaccination (an enquiry into the causes and effects of the variolae vaccinae, 1798). A sample of 23 people was infected with cowpox ($n = 23$). The probability of contacting smallpox when innoculated with the virus was some 90 per cent ($p = 0.9$), but none of the previously vaccinated 23 people did in fact contract smallpox ($r = 0$). The binomial probability of such an event occurring is exceedingly small, and the observations are therefore definitely not random.

A further binomial problem, this time with relevance to clinical trials, is stated in Table 5.4.

The method of solution and answer to the problem are given in Table 5.5.

The relevant binomial probability is therefore 0.094 or 9.4 per cent, that is, 94 chances per 1 000 experiments that the results are random — each experiment consisting of six matched pairs.

Table 5.4
Description of a
binomial problem

Experiment	Testing whether one of two drugs, *A* or *B* is more *effective*. Pairs of patients matched for sex and age are placed in the trial and one of each pair is randomly assigned to drug *A* or *B*.
Problem?	There are 6 matched pairs and in 5 cases drug *A* was found to be more *effective* than drug *B*. Is this result likely to have occurred quite randomly? — or can it be assumed that there is a *real* difference between *A* and *B*?
No. of trials, n	$n = 6$. In this problem, n will equal the number of matched pairs, each pair being regarded as a single experiment.
Probability of success, p	What do we choose for p, the probability that *A* is more effective than *B*? Since we have no concrete evidence beforehand, choose in the first instance $p = 0.5$, $(1 - p) = 0.5$. That is, it is equally likely either that *A* is more effective than *B* or that *B* is more effective than *A*.

Table 5.5
Calculation of a
binomial probability

Value of r the number of successes (i.e. *A* more effective than *B*)	^nC_r	p^r where $p = 0.5$	$(1 - p)^{n-r}$ where $n = 6$	Binomial probability from Formula 5.3
0	1			
1	6			
2	15			
3	20			
4	15			
5	6	$(\frac{1}{2})^5 = 1/32$	$(\frac{1}{2})^1 = \frac{1}{2}$	3/32 = 0.094
6	1			

The case when there are five successes is the case of interest in this problem

We now pass to the subject of *statistical significance*, which will be covered in Chapter 6. It is the *investigator who must fix the value of the limiting probability level*. This is the level below which he will accept that the results were *not* obtained by chance, i.e were *not* random. For this example, Tables 5.4 and 5.5 assume that the level fixed was 0.10. Since 0.094 is less than 0.10, he would accept that *A* is a more effective treatment than *B*. A stricter criterion would be the 0.05 level — and if this were chosen, since 0.094 is greater than 0.05, he would have to accept that no difference had been demonstrated between *A* and *B* at the 0.05 level. The investigators follow-up step would then be to repeat the experiment with a greater number of matched pairs, that is, n greater than 6, in the hope of a clearer answer.

The Normal Approximation to the Binomial

Figure 5.2 is a *binomial probability distribution* when $n = 3$ and $p = 3/5$ ($np = 1.8$). As the value of n increases, so will the range of *r*-values, and the distribution takes on a bell-shaped pattern, that can be approximated to a *normal* probability distribution under certain circumstances which are usually taken to be:

> Large n and 'not too small' p, where the product np is greater than 5

The advantage of this normal approximation to the binomial is that the standard tables available for the normal curve may be used for binomial problems when np is greater than 5.

Figure 5.2
Binomial probabilities

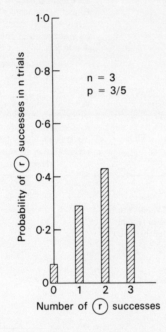

Mean and Standard Deviation of the Binomial Distribution

Formula 5.4
Formula 5.5

Mean, $\mu = np$
Standard deviation, $\sigma = \sqrt{n \cdot p \cdot q}$
  where $q = (1 - p)$

The Poisson Distribution

The *Poisson* distribution is a distribution in its own right, but it is also a limiting form of the *binomial* distribution.

A binomial distribution may be imagined in which the probability of *success*, p, is very nearly *equal to 1*, and the probability of *failure* $(1 - p)$ is very nearly *equal to 0*, so that the product $n \cdot (1 - p)$ is small. If we also have a large number, n, of experiments, then $(n - r)$ can be assumed to be equal to n since r will be negligible compared with n. Under these conditions, the formula for the binomial probabilities becomes:

Formula 5.6
Poisson probability

$$e^{-\mu} \cdot \frac{\mu^r}{r!}$$

which is known as the *Poisson distribution*. It is defined entirely by one constant, μ, which is the *mean* of the distribution. The *standard deviation* is also equal to μ. The e in the formula is the exponential encountered earlier in Formula 3.1.

No. of occurrences (r)	Formula for Poisson Probability	Poisson Probabilities for different values of μ		
		$\mu = 0.5$	$\mu = 1$	$\mu = 5$
0	$e^{-\mu}$	0.607	0.368	0.007
1	$\mu \cdot e^{-\mu}$	0.303	0.368	0.034
2	$(0.5) \cdot \mu^2 \cdot e^{-\mu}$	0.076	0.184	0.084
3	$(0.17) \cdot \mu^3 \cdot e^{-\mu}$	0.013	0.061	0.140
4	$(0.042) \cdot \mu^4 \cdot e^{-\mu}$	0.002	0.015	0.174
5	$(0.0083) \cdot \mu^5 \cdot e^{-\mu}$	0.000	0.003	0.174

Table 5.6 quotes some Poisson probabilities calculated using Formula 5.6, and it is noted that for μ greater than 25, the *normal* curve approximates to the Poisson distribution.

The Poisson distribution is applied whenever there is a large number of persons at risk, but the probability of an event occurring is very small. The classic example for the Poisson distribution is the distribution of the number of cavalrymen kicked to death in 10 Prussian Army Corps over a period of 20 years (Bortkiewiecz, T. 1898, Das Gesetz der kleinen Zahlen). This data is displayed in Table 5.7 and shows a close agreement between observation and theory. The experiment is to observe the number of deaths in a year in a single cavalry corps. The total number of deaths observed was 123 and the total number of experiments was 200, that is, 10 corps each observed for 20 separate years. The mean of the Poisson distribution is therefore $\mu = 123/200 = 0.61$. The theoretical Poisson frequencies for a given number of deaths, is obtained by multiplication of the *total number of experiments*, 200 in this case, and the *Poisson probability* given in Formula 5.6.

Actual No. of deaths per cavalry corps	Observed frequency	Poisson frequency when $\mu = 0.61$
0	109	108.7
1	65	66.3
2	22	20.2
3	3	4.1
4	1	0.6
5	0	0.01

Events for which Poisson probabilities may be calculated can occur either in time or in space. An example of a distribution in time is that of radioactive decay. In the medical use of radioactive isotopes for therapy and diagnosis, the radioactivity of a sample is estimated using a Geiger counter or more sophisticated instrumentation. The count rate distribution will be Poisson, and the probability of observing a given number of counts N when, on the average 20 counts are observed in a particular interval, will be given by the Poisson distribution with $\mu = 20$, and $r = N$. An example of a distribution in space is the distribution of red cells, white cells and platelets on the slide of a haemocytometer.

The data in the examples quoted above can all be fitted by Poisson probabilities. One example of a large population at risk, and a small probability of the occurrence of an event, is the incidence of a condition such as phocomelia. Let us suppose that in five large maternity units from 1940–1965 there was one reported case of phocomelia every two years, whereas in the years 1966–1968, during the use of thalidomide, the numbers of cases observed were 2, 5 and 4 in the respective years. $\mu = 0.5$ for the Poisson distribution describing the incidence of phocomelia. Table 5.8 gives the Poisson probabilities that for $\mu = 0.5$, two, five and four cases would occur in a given year, see Table 5.6.

Table 5.8
Phocomelia — a
Poisson problem

Year	No. of phocomelia cases	Theoretical Poisson probability of occurrence
1966	2	7.6 chances in 100
1967	5	0.02 chances in 100
1968	4	1.3　chances in 100

When testing data to see if the observations can be explained using the Poisson distribution, a certain numerical value, P, for the *number of chances in 100*, must be regarded as a critical probability. If the theoretical probability, such as that in Table 5.8, falls *below P*, then the observations are unlikely to have occurred randomly, and some external factor must be present. P is usually taken to be *5 chances in 100*. The choice of P will be discussed in Chapter 6 in more detail. From Table 5.8 it is seen that the theoretical chances of the observations which occurred in 1967 and 1968 being random are much less than 5 per 100. This is strong evidence that there is some predisposing factor causing the increase in the number of phocomelia cases.

Chapter 6

Statistical Significance

Introduction

In the example of Table 5.4 used to discuss binomial probabilities, the first mention was made of *significance* and *probability levels* ($P = 0.05$ and $P = 0.10$), which needed to be *set by the investigator*. The last four words of the previous sentence are very important, because they signify the fact that statistical techniques involving mathematical formulae cannot be used blindly without due thought. Statistics are not a cosmetic to be applied to give apparent credence to doubtful data! Not only does the correct significance test for a particular problem have to be chosen, but also the critical *probability level* at which we accept or reject the hypothesis under consideration. The choice of the probability level should be determined by the catastrophes that would happen if we are too optimistic or too pessimistic in analysing the data. In a clinical context this may be the acceptance of treatment A as the better treatment, when the better is really treatment B. The discussion in this chapter is intended to ensure that the general principles are understood and terminology explained. Chapter 7 and 8 will describe specific significance tests.

The Null Hypothesis

The starting point in the practical use of a test for significance is the statement of the *null hypothesis*, usually denoted by H_0. *Alternative hypotheses*, of which there may be one or more, can be denoted H_1, H_2, ... etc. A *hypothesis* is a set of assumptions expressed in a coherent manner about observable phenomena.

Examples of null hypotheses are given in Table 6.1.

Table 6.1
Four null hypotheses

There is no difference between:		
(*a*) The age distribution of a group of patients	*and*	a normal distribution
(*b*) The incidence of road accidents on a certain motorway	*and*	a random pattern
(*c*) The chance of having cancer of the lung subsequent to having cancer of the larynx	*and*	the chance of having cancer of the lung in the general population
(*d*) The effect of treatment A	*and*	The effect of treatment B

Consider null hypothesis (*d*) in Table 6.1 which is being investigated in a clinical trial. A description of the situation is given in Figure 6.1.

We have two alternatives with respect to the null hypothesis, rejection or acceptance, our choice being determined by the probability level we have decided upon. The consequences of these two courses of action are:

CONSEQUENCES

If we accept H_0, *the consequence → prolonging the trial?*

If we reject H_0, *the consequence → the discontinuation of one treatment in preference to another*

Figure 6.1
Hypothesis testing

Treatment A   Treatment B

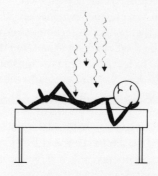
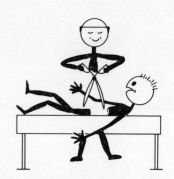

<u>Null</u> H_0 = there is <u>no difference</u> between treatment A and treatment B

<u>Alternative</u> hypotheses, H_1 = there is a difference between A and B, and <u>A is better</u>

H_2 = there is a difference between A and B, and <u>B is better</u>

The problem is to minimise the risks of making decisions which could lead to disastrous consequences. One such catastrophe would be to *accept that H_1 is true* on the basis of too little information and an insufficiently stringent critical level of probability, when reality was that hypothesis H_2 is correct. The two risks, related to (i) accepting H_0 or (ii) rejecting H_0, have to be *balanced* against each other. The relationship between the two types of risk will be discussed later after first summarising below what is meant *statistically* by the word *acceptance* when it refers to a hypothesis. It does *not* imply a future act of blind faith! It is important to understand this concept of *statistical acceptance*, and the fact that there is always some room for

It is up to the investigator to decide that the probability of occurrence is so small that it can be disregarded. The decision is not made by reference to a standard textbook.

THE 'DECEASED' LEFT FUNERAL, SWEARING

Caracas, October 2

When grave-diggers shovelled the first spadefuls of earth into a grave in the village cemetery at Pecaya, Venezuela, the "dead" man, Roberto Rodriguez, who had collapsed after a heart attack, burst open the lid of the coffin, scrambled out of the grave, and ran home shouting and swearing.

His mother-in-law, who was standing at the graveside, dropped dead from shock. She will be buried in the grave prepared for her son-in-law, after doctors have made absolutely certain there is no mistake this time.—Reuter.

doubt, since all acceptance and rejection statements are *qualified* by the description 'at a probability level of . . . ' (e.g. $P = 0.05$). Even what might appear to be the most unlikely of events will have a finite chance of occurrence albeit very small.

Acceptance of a null hypothesis
If H_0 has not been rejected at a given level of probability then we must assume that it has been *accepted*. However, this really implies *not proven* — because we are working in terms of probability. What *acceptance* means is that *if the hypothesis is in fact false, then the experiment was not able to detect it at the established level of significance.*

Alpha and Beta Risks

DEFINITIONS   The procedure in significance testing is to first formulate the null hypothesis, H_0, rather than an alternative hypothesis, H_1 or H_2 and then to test this null hypothesis. There are two types of error called *type I error* and *type II error*, which describe two different kinds of *catastrophe* which could occur if the critical level of probability for the test is too large, that is the test is not stringent enough. The *risk* is the probability of actually making one of these kinds of mistake, Table 6.2.

Table 6.2
Error types, the null hypothesis and α and β risks

Error	Definition of error type	Associated risk
Type I	Wrongly rejecting H_0 when H_0 is true	Probability [Type I error] $= \alpha$
Type II	Wrongly accepting H_0 when H_0 is false	Probability [Type II error] $= \beta$

The β-risk is a function of an alternative hypothesis, and since H_0 is false, H_1 or H_2 must be true. The probability $[1 - \beta]$ is defined as the *power of the test* of the hypothesis H_0 against an alternative hypothesis.

The α-risk is the chance of wrongly rejecting H_0 and acting upon the premise *that at the α-level there is a difference.* The consequence of this in treatment evaluation for example, is *the discontinuation of one particular treatment* in preference to another.

The β-risk is the chance of wrongly accepting the null hypothesis when it is false. We then accept *that there is no difference.* The consequence which follows could be either *that we attempt further investigations* or *discontinue the trial* without reaching any conclusion as to whether one treatment is better than the other.

α *and β-risks are related*, they are *not independent* of each other. If the α-risk is increased, then the β-risk is decreased, and vice-versa. In order to clarify the concepts of α and β risks, and their interrelation, schematic diagrams will now be introduced.

In Figure 3.7, and Table 3.2 a *visual representation* of probability was given using a normal curve, and a total probability of 1 was equated to the whole area beneath the curve. Probabilities of occurrence of an event between standard deviation limits such as ± 1 σ were given in terms of a percentage chance. In an example in Chapter 4 the event of interest was a male height of 183 cm. Not all events can be described by a normal probability distribution, some are lognormal for instance, and thus the probability distribution of Figure 6.2 is to be considered only as an example of a distribution.

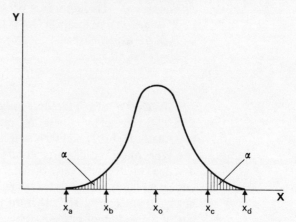

Figure 6.2
Probability distribution
centred on x_0

The probability distribution of Figure 6.2 is symmetrical about x_0. We will define our *null hypothesis*, H_0, to be that:

> *there is no difference between an observed distribution of male heights, and the probability distribution in Figure 6.2 which is centred on x_0*

We have to talk about *distributions* rather than *single valued* observations and expectations, since in practice there will be a *spread* of expected values. The null hypothesis is *not* merely that the observation = x_0, it *must* be that *the observed distribution = the distribution centred on x_0.*

Having accepted that Figure 6.2 represents probability, we can now answer a few questions in terms of the diagram.

Question 1 What is the probability of an observation lying in the range x_a to x_b?

Answer The area under the curve between the values of x_a and x_b on the x-axis which has been shaded and denoted by α. [The total area under the curve is equal to 1.]

Question 2 What is the probability of an observation lying in the range x_c to x_d where $(x_b - x_a) = (x_d - x_c)$?

Answer The area under the curve between the values of x_c and x_d on the x-axis. This has also been shaded and called α.

The *α-risk* is the chance of wrongly rejecting H_0 when it is true, Table 6.3. When H_0 is true, then Figure 6.2 is a true representation of the frequency distribution of x. We wish to minimise the α-risk, and so we can choose to say that if an observed value of x falls towards the ends of the curve in Figure 6.2 within the shaded areas, then we will reject H_0. There is only a small probability (i.e. α) of such an event happening because most of the observations will fall beneath the central part of the curve.

$P = 0.05$

It is now up to the investigator to fix a numerical value for α. By convention, this is usually 0.05, 0.01 or 0.10, but it *must* (i) depend upon the judgement of the investigator, and (ii) it must be decided *before* the trial is undertaken. The α-risk is a probability and the notation is usually $P = \ldots$. If the α-risk is set at the $P = 0.05$ level of significance, then the investigator has accepted the risk that there are *five false results* in every hundred. That is, there are five chances in a hundred of finding a so-called *difference* when no such difference really exists.

One-tailed and Two-tailed Tests

In Figure 6.2 there are two shaded *tail* areas labelled α. The one on the left-hand end of the x-axis is *less than x_0* and the one on the right hand end of the x-axis is *greater than x_0*. A *one-tailed test* is that in which only *one* of the shaded areas in Figure 6.2 is used. That is, if the investigator is only interested in:

observations being significantly *less* than those of the x_0 distribution

or only in

observations being significantly *greater* than those of the x_0 distribution.

A one-tailed, $P = 0.05$, test would therefore have an α corresponding to $P = 0.05$ at one or other end of the x_0 distribution.

A *two-tailed test* is that in which *both* of the shaded areas in Figure 6.2 are used, when the investigator is interested in observations being significantly *less* or observations being significantly *greater* than those of the x_0 distribution. For a two-tailed test one might have either both α-risks corresponding to $P = 0.05$, where $2\alpha = 0.10$ which corresponds to ten false results in every hundred; or both α risks corresponding to $P = 0.025$, where $2\alpha = 0.05$ which corresponds to 5 false results in every hundred.

If two alternative treatment techniques A and B, Figure 6.1, are being investigated, then we would like to know if A *is better than* B or if B *is better than* A. This is a *two-tailed test* situation. If, however, A and B are drug treatments and B is a placebo, then we are usually only interested in the knowledge of whether A *is better than* B and this is a *one-tailed test* situation.

Beta Risk

In Figure 6.2 we already have a visual representation of the probability distribution centred on x_0. In Figure 6.3 two probability distributions are shown, the first one centred on x_0 as in Figure 6.2

and the second on a different value of x, equal to x_1. It can be seen that the two distributions overlap and that the *cross-over point* for the two curves is near $x = x_c$. The null hypothesis has already been defined so let us choose an *alternative* hypothesis, H_1, which states that 'the observed distribution of male heights is *not* that centred on x_0, but rather one centred on x_1'.

Figure 6.3
Two probability distributions
centred on x_0 and x_1

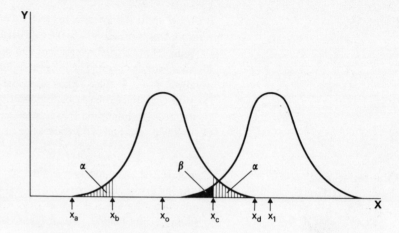

The *β-risk*, Table 6.2 is the chance of wrongly accepting the null hypothesis H_0 when it is false. If the null hypothesis *is* false, then some other hypothesis must be the correct one, and *what should have happened* is that the alternative hypothesis H_1 should have been accepted. We are assuming for simplicity in this example that there is *only* one alternative hypothesis, H_1, and not a series $H_1, H_2, \ldots$ one of which is the correct one. Looking at the central portion of Figure 6.3 where the two curves overlap, there are two shaded areas, α to the right of x_c and β to the left of x_c. The following comments can now be made.

1. Since we are discussing *wrongly accepting H_0*, the observation x (which for example may be a measurement of height), must lie between x_b and x_c since this is the region of acceptance. The regions of rejection of H_0 are from x_a to x_b, and from x_c to x_d, namely the regions labelled α.

2. If, however, H_0 is false and H_1 is true, then it can be imagined that the observed value of x we are considering has fallen into that small overlap region labelled β in Figure 6.3, which belongs to both probability distributions. We will then assume, erroneously, that it belongs to the x_0 distribution, and therefore *wrongly accept H_0*, when in fact it belongs to the x_1 distribution and we should have rejected H_0 and accepted H_1. It is the risk of this type of error occurring that is specified by the β risk.

3. It is the investigator who sets the limits for α and β, the x_b and the x_c values, and it can be seen from the centre of Figure 6.3 that if α is reduced and limit x_c moved towards the right, then since the

two curves remain stationary, the area β to the left of x_c will increase. The reverse would occur if limit x_c were moved towards the left.

Standard Deviation and Standard Error

Standard deviation, σ, has been defined for a set of observations and two alternative methods of calculating σ have been previously given. Figure 3.7 and Table 3.2 have also elaborated on the meaning of σ for the normal and lognormal distributions.

Let us assume that we have a trial with two groups of patients, A and B, and that we have measured a certain quantity Y for each group, which varies with a quantity X. For example, Y might be the fraction surviving to a given time (X) after treatment. This is illustrated in Figure 6.4 in which twice the associated standard deviation, $\pm 2\sigma$, is plotted as a vertical bar for each point graphed. The information contained on the graph is therefore ($[Y \pm 2\sigma]$; X) for all points. We will further assume that if the trial were repeated many times, then the spread of values for any of the points in Figure 6.4 would follow a normal probability distribution, and if a plotted point in Figure 6.4 was the true mean value of Y for a given X-value, some 95 per cent of all Y-values for the given X would lie within the limits of the error bar.

Figure 6.4
Graph with error bars

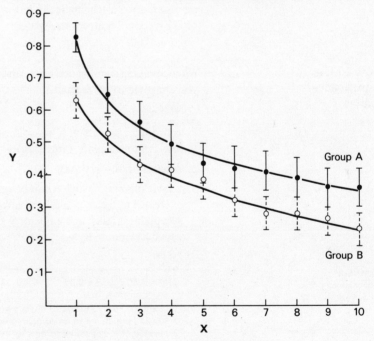

If there is no overlap of any of the 2σ error bars for groups A and B then this indicates that the Y-values are significantly different for the two groups at the $P = 0.05$ level of significance. If, however, for a single X-value, the 2σ error bars overlap, then this indicates that there is no significant difference, $P = 0.05$, in Y- values between groups A and B *for that particular X-value.* In Figure 6.4, if X represents years subsequent to treatment and Y represents the corresponding survival fraction,

$[Y = 1.0$ when $X = 0]$, then the graph indicates that there is no significant difference, $P = 0.05$, in survival results at $X = 5$ years. Drawing graphs and judging error bars *by eye*, is however, no substitute for testing the null hypothesis *there is no difference between the results for groups A and B* using the formal statistical tests of significance, (see Chapters 7 and 8).

Standard error is a special type of *standard deviation* which is the standard deviation of the *mean* of a series of observations. An important theorem in statistics is the *Central Limit Theorem* which states:

> *If a random sample of size n, is drawn from any population with mean μ and standard deviation σ, then as n increases, the distribution of* $\dfrac{\bar{x} - \mu}{\sigma/\sqrt{n}}$ *approaches the standard normal distribution*

This theorem is important because the sample may be drawn from *any* population, *not* just a normal population. $\bar{x}$ is a mean value from a series of observations, and the standard normal distribution referred to above is the *distribution of means*. The *grand mean* or *mean of means* is μ and the standard deviation of this μ is $\sigma/\sqrt{n}$. These statements are shown schematically in Figure 6.5. The quantity x may be blood pressure, temperature, pulse rate, . . . etc.

How to Use Significance Tables

When applying significance tests, first ensure that the particular test you are going to use is valid.

You will have:

1. A formula into which observations, expressed as numbers, can be inserted to calculate a *test statistic*.

2. A series of observations.

3. A table of values which *could* be obtained from the formula expressed in terms of a critical level of probability, P (the acceptable α risk); and a quantity known as *degrees of freedom* which is denoted by ν.

Table 6.3
Significance table
for a hypothetical
Γ-test

$P = 0.10$	$P = 0.05$	$P = 0.01$
$\nu = 1$	Table of critical values of a test statistic	
$\nu = 2$	(say Γ) which are to be compared with	
$\nu = 3$	a value of Γ calculated using a formula,	
$\nu = 4$	see Note 1 above.	
$\nu = 5$		
etc.		

Figure 6.5
Standard deviation and
standard error

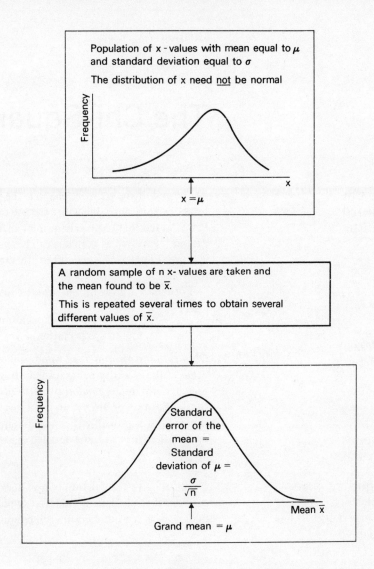

When the test statistic, Γ, has been calculated, the number of
degrees of freedom determined (this will be dealt with in Chapters 7
and 8 for the different tests), and the level of significance chosen, you
will (i) look up the critical value of Γ from Table 6.3 which corresponds
to the relevant value of ν and the chosen value of P, (ii) compare the
critical value of Γ with the calculated value of Γ.

If Γ *is less than critical* Γ, then you conclude that *there is no
significant difference*, at the *P-probability level.*

If Γ *is greater than critical* Γ then you conclude that *there is
a significant difference*, at the *P-probability level.*

The Chi-Squared Test

The Chi-Squared Statistic, χ^2

At the end of the previous chapter, the general procedure for applying tests of significance, including the use of significance tables, was given. It was stated that the mechanism involved a formula into which observations, expressed as numbers can be inserted to calculate a *test statistic*. For the chi-squared test, this test statistic is χ^2, for the *t*-test it is *t* and for the F-test it is F.

Formula 7.1 gives the *chi-squared* test statistic where

Formula 7.1 Chi-squared statistic

$$\chi^2 = \frac{(\text{observation} - \text{expectation})^2}{(\text{expectation})}$$

Observation is the *observed value*, and *expectation* is the *expected value* of the quantity being studied. In some cases the test is to see if the observations are *randomly distributed* and in others to test whether the distribution of observations follows a definite pattern. The chi-squared test is probably the most frequently used significance test in medical statistics and so a detailed discussion of its applications will be given.

Frequency Tables — Observed and Expected

To illustrate the calculation of a χ^2 test statistic using Formula 7.1, consider first the data in Table 7.1, which consists of five columns of figures, with ten numbers in each column.

Table 7.1 χ^2 test data

O	E	(O − E)	(O − E)^2	$\chi^2 = (O − E)^2/E$
18	25	−7	49	2.0
31	25	6	36	1.4
29	25	4	16	0.6
36	25	11	121	4.8
17	25	−8	64	2.6
20	25	−5	25	1.0
20	25	−5	25	1.0
35	25	10	100	4.0
14	25	−11	121	4.8
30	25	5	25	1.0

The sum of the ten individual values of χ^2 is 23.2 and this is denoted by $\Sigma\chi^2$.

There are ten observations, all quoted in the first column, of a quantity which is expected to have a value equal to 25, thus the null hypothesis is that the 'true' value of our experimental observation is equal to 25.

Corresponding expected values are quoted in the second column. The numerator of the fraction in Formula 7.1 is $(O - E)^2$, and the first step required is therefore to calculate $(O - E)$, which is given in the third column, preparatory to calculating $(O - E)^2$, which is given in the fourth column. The value of χ^2 for each individual observation is then obtained by dividing the entry in the fourth column by the entry in the second column. These values of χ^2 are given in the fifth and final column. The test statistic is the summation of *all* the individual χ^2 values.

If prior to the calculation we have fixed the critical level of probability at $P = 0.05$, only the number of degrees of freedom v are required before the significance table for the χ^2 test can be used. For a frequency table of the type in Table 7.1, the *degrees of freedom* equal the total number of pairs of O and E values *minus one*. Thus, if there are n pairs of O and E values,

Formula 7.2
Degrees of freedom

$$v = [n - 1]$$

Finally, we need a significance table of the type described in Table 6.3 in the previous chapter. Table 7.2 is the relevant table.

Table 7.2
Critical values of χ^2 for different degrees of freedom (v) and probability levels ($P = 0.05$, 0.01)

	$P = 0.05$	$P = 0.01$
$v = 1$	3.84	6.64
$v = 2$	5.99	9.21
$v = 3$	7.82	11.34
$v = 4$	9.49	13.28
$v = 5$	11.07	15.09
$v = 6$	12.59	16.81
$v = 7$	14.07	18.48
$v = 8$	15.51	20.09
$v = 9$	16.92	21.67
$v = 10$	18.31	23.21

The *null hypothesis*, H_0, which is being tested is that there is no difference between observation (O) and expectation (E) at the $P = 0.05$ level of probability. The information we have at our disposal to test H_0 is:

(a) $\Sigma\chi^2$ from Formula 7.1 which is 23.2.
(b) The number of degrees of freedom, $v = [10 - 1] = 9$.
(c) The critical value of χ^2 from Table 7.2 for $v = 9$ and $P = 0.05$, which is 16.92.

The final step in the testing procedure is to note that since 23.2 is greater than 16.92, we must conclude that there *is* a significant difference (at $P = 0.05$ level) between O and E values. An alternative terminology for *probability level*, $P = 0.05$ is 95 per cent *confidence level*. P is given as a *decimal* less than 1 and confidence level is given as a *percentage* equal to $[100 \times (1 - P)]$.

Consider the data in Table 7.4. The pattern of the two sexes in families is an example of a binomial situation, Chapter 5, since there are only two possibilities and the sex of a child is independent of the sex of earlier children in a family. If we assume that the chance of a

Table 7.3
Rejection and
acceptance of the
null hypothesis

CALCULATION	CONCLUSION
If the calculated $\Sigma\chi^2$ is *greater* than the critical value of χ^2.	We accept that there is a significant difference between O and E at the chosen level of probability, *P*, and we *reject the null hypothesis, H_0*.
If the calculated $\Sigma\chi^2$ is *less* than the critical value of χ^2.	We cannot reject, H_0, and instead, say that at the chosen level of probability, *P*, that *if* there is in fact a difference between O and E, we cannot detect it at this probability level, *P*.

boy is 0.5 and the chance of a girl is 0.5, then the binomial probability $\beta = 0.5$. The χ^2 test may be used to test whether the data of Table 7.4 is in agreement with this hypothesis at the $P = 0.05$ probability level, or whether some unknown factor in this family has influenced the sex ratio to such an extent that there is not an equal chance for boys and girls.

The observed values (O) for the χ^2 test are those given in Table 7.4, and the expected values (E) are calculated by multiplying the [total number of families] by the [binomial probability from Formula 5.3].

Table 7.4

Genealogical data
for use in a binomial
calculation

First 2 children born in a family		First 3 children born in a family	
2 boys	14	3 boys	7
1 boy + 1 girl	28	2 boys + 1 girl	13
2 girls	8	1 boy + 2 girls	11
		3 girls	1
Total No. of families =	50	Total No. of families =	32

Data from a family tree of a male emigrant (one of four brothers) to New Zealand in 1867 (b. 1843, m. 1878, d. 1908) with a complete follow-up for 1843–1973. It contains 180 members including 15 families of 4 or more children.

Summation of χ^2 has for this example been calculated below, where β denotes the binomial probability.

(a) *For the first 2 children born in a family*

	β	E	O	$\chi^2 = (O - E)^2/E$
2b	0.25	12.5	14	0.2
1b + 1g	0.50	25	28	0.4
2g	0.28	12.5	8	1.6

$\Sigma\chi^2 = 2.2$, No. of degrees of freedom, $\nu = (3 - 1) = 2$

(b) *For the first 3 children born in a family*

	β	E	O	$\chi^2 = (O-E)^2/E$
3b	0.125	4	7	2.3
2b + 1g	0.375	12	13	0.1
1b + 2g	0.375	12	11	0.1
3g	0.125	4	1	2.3

$\Sigma\chi^2 = 4.8$, No. of degrees of freedom, $v = (4-1) = 3$

From Table 7.2 it is seen that for $P = 0.05$, the critical value of χ^2 for $v = 2$ is 5.99 and for $v = 3$ is 7.82. In both cases above, the calculated $\Sigma\chi^2$ is therefore *less than* the critical value of χ^2, and we therefore accept the null hypothesis which states that there is no difference at the $P = 0.05$ level between the observations, and those expected using binomial theory.

Curve Fitting

Curve fitting problems involve a null hypothesis, H_0, of the form *there is no difference between the distribution of observed values and the distribution of the expected values calculated from a given mathematical formula*. Returning to Figure 3.4 it is noted that the diagram contains a series of observed frequencies for survival times of cancer patients in the form of a histogram. The curve superimposed on the histogram is a theoretical curve from which expected frequencies can be calculated. The problem is to decide whether at the $P = 0.05$ probability level, we can *accept H_0*, showing that the theoretical curve *is* a good approximation to the observed distribution.

Table 7.5 lists the observed and expected frequency values for eleven survival time intervals, and the expected values have been calculated using the lognormal curve whose formula is

$$Y = \frac{1}{S\sqrt{2\pi}} \cdot \frac{1}{T} \cdot e^{-\frac{1}{2}\frac{[(\log_e T) - M]^2}{S^2}}$$

and has previously been given as Formula 3.4. In the lognormal formula there are two unknown *variable parameters*, the mean logtime, M, and the standard deviation, S, both of which can be estimated using log-probability graph paper as described in Chapter 3. The need to make estimates of parameters in a formula, prior to computing $\Sigma\chi^2$, is taken into account when calculating the number of degrees of freedom, v, to be used in the test. In the examples in Tables 7.1 and 7.4 it was $(n - 1)$, Formula 7.2, where n = the number of pairs of O and E values. The formula for calculating the degrees of freedom for curve fitting problems is

Formula 7.3
Degrees of freedom

$$v = [n - \frac{\text{Number of formula parameters which have to be estimated,}}{} - 1]$$

For the example of Table 7.5, the number of lognormal parameters which have to be estimated equals 2 and, hence, the degrees of freedom $\nu = (11 - 2 - 1) = 8$. From Table 7.2, the critical value of χ^2 equals 15.51 for $P = 0.05$ and $\nu = 8$. Since the calculated $\Sigma\chi^2 = 12.4$ is less than 15.51, we do *not reject* the null hypothesis, and we can assume that the observed distribution of survival times can be represented by a lognormal curve.

Survival Time range in years (T)	O	E
$0-\frac{1}{2}$	56	57.1
$\frac{1}{2}-1$	107	98.1
$1-2$	155	146.7
$2-3$	78	87.9
$3-4$	62	54.6
$4-6$	50	60.1
$6-8$	30	29.8
$8-10$	27	16.5
$10-12$	10	9.9
$12-14$	5	6.3
$14-16$	3	4.2

$\Sigma\chi^2 = 12.4$, No. of degrees of freedom, $\nu = (11 - 3) = 8$

The 2 x 2 Contingency Table

A 2 x 2 contingency table is used when a series of observations can be grouped according to two criteria, with each criteria having two levels. This is illustrated in Table 7.6. The problem to be solved is whether the two criteria of interest are independent of each other. For example, whether treatment results at patient follow-up are independent of the treatment!

Criterion	Levels
Patient follow-up	1 Alive 2 Dead
Treatment	1 Type A 2 Type B
Diet	1 Diet A 2 Diet B
Sex	1 Male 2 Female
Age group	1 Group A 2 Group B

To illustrate the method, consider a hypothetical group of 20 patients, 11 of whom had been treated using drug A and the remaining 9 treated using drug B. There were 5 responders in the drug A group and 2 responders in the drug B group. The two criteria are therefore *treatment* with the two levels as (1) drug A, and (2) drug B; and *response* with the two levels as (1) response, (2) no response. The contingency table is drawn up below:

Table 7.7
2 x 2 contingency
table containing the
observed numbers

	RESPONSE		Row Totals
TREATMENT	Some	None	
Drug A	5	6	11
Drug B	2	7	9
Column totals	7	13	Grand total = 20

The numbers in Table 7.7 are *observed* values. The *expected* values for the contingency table χ^2-test are calculated using the Formula 7.4, as shown in Table 7.8. and the calculation of $\Sigma\chi^2$ is as shown in Table 7.9.

Formula 7.4
Contingency table
expected values

$$\text{Expected value} = \frac{(\text{row total} \times \text{column total})}{\text{grand total}}$$

Table 7.8
2 x 2 contingency
table containing the
expected numbers

	RESPONSE		Row totals
TREATMENT	Some	None	
Drug A	$\dfrac{11 \times 7}{20}$	$\dfrac{11 \times 13}{20}$	11
Drug B	$\dfrac{9 \times 7}{20}$	$\dfrac{9 \times 13}{20}$	9
Column totals	7	13	Grand total = 20

→ WHICH EQUALS →

3.9	7.2
3.2	5.9

Table 7.9
Calculation of $\Sigma\chi^2$

O	E	$\chi^2 = (O - E)^2 / E$
5	3.9	0.3
6	7.2	0.2
2	3.2	0.5
7	5.9	0.2

$\Sigma\chi^2 = 1.2$ and the number of degrees of freedom for a 2 x 2 contingency table are $v = 1$.

Since the calculated $\Sigma\chi^2$ of 1.2 is less than the critical value of χ^2, Table 7.2, for $P = 0.05$ and $v = 1$, which is 3.84, we do *not reject* the null hypothesis, and we accept that for the data available the results have shown, at the $P = 0.05$ level of probability, that treatment and response are independent of each other, and hence one drug is not producing significantly more responses than the other.

The example of Tables 7.7 to 7.9 is hypothetical data with simple numbers to illustrate the method. A practical example is given below, using exactly the same method of calculation. The data has been taken from De Lorenzo, *et al.*, *Lancet*, **1**, 669, (1974) and is relevant to the Naples cholera epidemic of 1973. The objective of the test is to determine whether consumption of raw mussels was a significant factor in the cause of the outbreak of cholera. Data is available for a total of 911 persons admitted to hospital.

Table 7.10
Cholera epidemic data

CHOLERA INFECTION

	Infected	*Not* Infected	Row totals
Number who consumed raw mussels in preceding 5 days	41	89	130
Number who did *not* consume raw mussels	85	696	781
Column totals	126	785	Grand total = 911

(DIET)

The expected values are $\dfrac{18 \mid 112}{108 \mid 673}$ and the calculated $\Sigma\chi^2$ is 38.1.

This is far greater than the critical value of χ^2 for $\nu = 1$ and $P = 0.01$, which is 6.64, and we must therefore reject the null hypothesis and state that a raw mussel diet and cholera infection are dependent upon each other.

Two other examples in which the null hypothesis is rejected because the calculated $\Sigma\chi^2$ is greater than the critical value of χ^2 are:

(*a*) In a trial of *typhoid* inoculation (Leishman, 1909, *Journal of the Royal Army Medical Corps*, **12**, 163–7).

	No. developing typhoid	No. not developing typhoid
Inoculated	21	5452
Not Inoculated	187	6423

the calculated $\Sigma\chi^2$ is 106.

(*b*) In a trial of *penicillin* for *Staphylococcus aureus* infection in the mouse (Chain *et al.*, 1940 *Lancet*, **2**, 226–8) the calculated $\Sigma\chi^2$ is 37.3.

	No. of mice surviving	No. of mice dying
Treated	21	3
Not Treated	0	24

Finally, it is noted that the 2 x 2 contingency table is the simplest available, and that for a general table with more columns and rows, Formula 7.5 is required to calculate the required number of degrees of freedom.

Formula 7.5
Degrees of freedom
(contingency table)

$$\nu = (\text{No. of rows} - 1) \times (\text{No. of columns} - 1)$$

Chapter 8

Further Tests of Significance

The *t*-Test

There are two types of significance tests and they are described as *parametric* and *non-parametric*. For the parametric tests, certain conditions *should* exist for the population being tested. For non-parametric tests, no such conditions are laid down. The χ^2 test of Chapter 7 is non-parametric, but the *t*-test and F-test in this chapter are parametric. The *condition* which must hold before a *t*- or F-test can be used is that *the population from which the sample under observation is drawn, must be normally distributed.* That is, the population distribution can be fitted by a *normal curve.* In practice, however, for some tests the investigator is allowed a certain latitude and as long as the population is *approximately* normal, the test may be applied. In statistical terminology, it is said that the test is *robust* when we can accept approximate normality. The *t*-test is a robust test.

The *frequency distribution of means is normal*, Figure 6.5, and the *t-test* is the test of significance used to investigate the *difference in means* from two samples. The *t*-statistic is given in Formula 8.1.

Formula 8.1
t-statistic

$$ t = \frac{(\text{Difference in means})}{(\text{Standard error of the difference in means})} = \frac{(\bar{X}_1 - \bar{X}_2)}{\dfrac{S}{\sqrt{N}}} $$

$\bar{X}_1$ and $\bar{X}_2$ are the means of the two samples, N is the number of observations and S is the standard deviation of the quantity $(X_1 - X_2)$.

As an example of the calculation procedure, suppose that a hypothetical group of 4 patients have been treated and that a quantity of interest (e.g. weight, tumour size, . . .) was measured before and after treatment. The problem is to decide whether there has been any significant difference in this quantity during treatment.

Table 8.1
t-test data

Patient	Before treatment X_1	After treatment X_2
A	2	3
B	4	3
C	3	1
D	5	2

X (heading spanning Before and After treatment columns)

EXAMPLE USING PAIRED DATA Using the data in Table 8.1, the two sets of measurements, before and after treatment, are *paired* for each patient. The null hypothesis in the example is that there is no difference in quantity X before and after treatment, and that consequently both X_1 and X_2 are drawn from the same *normal* population and that $(X_1 - X_2)$ is normally distributed about a *mean equal to zero*.

Table 8.2 gives the arithmetic necessary for the *t*-test, Formula 8.1. Thus, $(\overline{X}_1 - \overline{X}_2) = (3.5 - 2.25) = 1.25$ which is the *numerator* of formula 8.1. Formula 2.2 may be used to calculate the standard deviation of $(X_1 - X_2)$.

Standard deviation:

$$S = \sqrt{\frac{\Sigma(X_1 - X_2)^2 - \frac{[\Sigma(X_1 - X_2)]^2}{N}}{(N-1)}}$$

$$S = \sqrt{\frac{1 - \frac{25}{4}}{3}} = 1.7$$

and $S/\sqrt{N}$ is the *denominator* of Formula 8.1.

$$S/\sqrt{N} = 0.85$$

Table 8.2
Calculations for a
paired *t*-test

	X_1	X_2	$(X_1 - X_2)$	$(X_1 - X_2)^2$	$X_1{}^2$	$X_2{}^2$
	2	3	−1	1	4	9
Individual	4	3	+1	1	16	9
values	3	1	+2	4	9	1
	5	2	+3	9	25	4
Sum of each column of figures	14	9	5	15	54	23
Mean values (divide by 4 in this example)	$\overline{X}_1 =$ 3.5	$\overline{X}_2 =$ 2.25				

The *t*-statistic is therefore equal to $(1.25/0.85) = 1.5$, and since there were 4 pairs of X_1 and X_2 values, the number of degrees of freedom, ν, is $(4 - 1) = 3$, Formula 8.2. Table 8.3 is the relevant table of critical values of the *t*-statistic. From this table, for $P = 0.05$ and $\nu = 3$, the critical value of $t = 3.18$. The calculated value of t is less than 3.18 and we therefore conclude that at the $P = 0.05$ level we *cannot reject H_0*, the null hypothesis. We must therefore assume that there is no detectable change *at this level of probability*, in the value of X before and after treatment.

Formula 8.2
Degrees of freedom

$$\nu = (\text{Number of pairs} - 1)$$

Table 8.3
Critical values of t
for different degrees
of freedom (v) and
probability levels
($P = 0.05$, 0.01). (t
may be either + or −)

	$P = 0.05$	$P = 0.01$
$v = 1$	12.71	63.66
$v = 2$	4.30	9.92
$v = 3$	3.18	5.84
$v = 4$	2.78	4.60
$v = 5$	2.57	4.03
$v = 6$	2.45	3.71
$v = 7$	2.36	3.50
$v = 8$	2.31	3.36
$v = 9$	2.26	3.25
$v = 10$	2.23	3.17
$v = \infty$	1.96	2.58

Two practical examples where the t-test, which is a test for a difference between means of groups, would be applicable are:

(*a*) Gain in weight after known pattern of protein intake.
(*b*) Duration of anaesthesia produced by two different drugs.

EXAMPLE USING UNPAIRED DATA   When the data is unpaired, the necessary formula is more complicated. To illustrate the calculation method, again use the data in Table 8.1 although this time the two sets of data cannot be matched for each patient name A, B, C and D. (The unpaired t-test would also be used if there were two *separate* groups of patients.) We cannot work *directly* with values of $(X_1 - X_2)$ as we did in Table 8.2 since the pairs are not matched. We can of course calculate $\bar{X}_1$ and $\bar{X}_2$, and find that $(\bar{X}_1 - \bar{X}_2) = 1.25$ in the same manner, but it is the standard error of the difference in means which has to be found by a different method.

Provided that the standard deviations of the two populations under test can be assumed to be equal, Formula 8.3 for the standard error of the difference in means is modified to become Formula 8.4, where $t = (\bar{X}_1 - \bar{X}_2)/\sigma$.

Formula 8.3
Standard error

$$\sigma = \frac{S}{\sqrt{N}}$$

Formula 8.4
Standard error

$$\sigma = \sqrt{\frac{[\Sigma X_1^2 - (\Sigma X_1)^2/N_1] + [\Sigma X_2^2 - (\Sigma X_2)^2/N_2]}{(N_1 - 1) + (N_2 - 1)} \times \left(\frac{1}{N_1} + \frac{1}{N_2}\right)}$$

For an *unpaired* t-test example there are four measurements ($N_1 = 4$) before treatment and four measurements ($N_2 = 4$) after treatment. The degrees of freedom are given by formula 8.5 which for our example gives $v = (4 - 1) + (4 - 1) = 6$.

Formula 8.5
Degrees of freedom

$$v = (N_1 - 1) + (N_2 - 1)$$

All the required [Σ . . .] are to be found in Table 8.2. Thus:

$$\sigma = \sqrt{\frac{[(54) - (14)^2/4] + [(23) - (9)^2/4]}{(4-1) + (4-1)} \times \left[\frac{1}{4} + \frac{1}{4}\right]} = \sqrt{0.645} = 0.8$$

and the t-statistic is calculated from Formula 8.1 as $t = 1.25/0.8 = 1.6$.

Previously for the *paired t*-test, we obtained $t = 1.5$, but this was for $\nu = 3$. Now we have $t = 1.6$ for $\nu = 6$. Having again chosen $P = 0.05$, we find from Table 8.3 that the critical value of t for $\nu = 6$ and $P = 0.05$ is 2.45. Since 1.6 is *less than* 2.45 we *cannot reject* H_0.

The F-Test

The *t-test* is used for testing *differences in means*, the *F-test* is used for testing *differences in variance*, where if variance is denoted by S^2, the standard deviation is S. Both tests contain the underlying assumption that the populations from which the samples are drawn are *normal*. The F-test, however, is not as *robust* as the *t*-test. The *F-statistic* is given by Formula 8.6.

Formula 8.6
F-statistic

$$F = \frac{\text{larger variance}}{\text{smaller variance}} = \frac{[S_1]^2}{[S_2]^2}$$

and the table of critical values of F is Table 8.4, where ν_1 is the degrees of freedom for the greater variance and ν_2 for the smaller variance.

Table 8.4
Critical values of F for different degrees of freedom (ν_1 and ν_2) and the probability level $P = 0.05$

	$\nu_1 = 1$	$\nu_1 = 2$	$\nu_1 = 3$	$\nu_1 = 4$	$\nu_1 = 5$
$\nu_2 = 1$	161	200	216	225	230
$\nu_2 = 2$	18.5	19.0	19.2	19.3	19.3
$\nu_2 = 3$	10.1	9.6	9.3	9.1	9.0
$\nu_2 = 4$	7.7	6.9	6.6	6.4	6.3
$\nu_2 = 5$	6.6	5.8	5.4	5.2	5.1
$\nu_2 = 6$	3.8	3.0	2.6	2.4	2.2

It must be noted that the F-test is a test for the comparison of two *independent* estimates of variance, and this condition *fails* if the observations in the two samples are *paired*.

The standard deviation S of a series of N observations can be calculated using Formula 2.2. *When* the F-test is required, S_1 and S_2 will be obtained in this manner and inserted into Formula 8.6. The calculated F-statistic is then compared with the critical value of F from Table 8.4.

The word 'when' is emphasised in the previous paragraph since the F-test is not required as often as the t-test since interest usually rests with a comparison of *position*, rather than with a comparison of *shape*.

As an example to illustrate the use of the F-test, consider ten patients placed in two different wards, whose systolic blood pressures are as given below:

Ward A patients: 170, 180, 160, 200, 180 mm Hg
Ward B patients: 210, 140, 160, 230, 150 mm Hg

The mean blood pressure of both groups is the same, equal to 178 mm Hg and the problem is to investigate whether the variability of the blood pressures is also the same for both groups so that they can be assumed to be from the same population; that is, with the same mean *and* standard deviation. If they do all come from the same population, then they may be paired with each other to assess the effect of an anti-hypertensive drug.

Using Formula 8.6 the F-statistic is equal to $(1575/225) = 7.0$; and from Table 8.4 for $\nu_1 = \nu_2 = 4$ degrees of freedom, and $P = 0.05$, the critical value of F is 6.4. Since 7.0 is greater than 6.4, we reject the null hypothesis *that both groups of patients are from the same population* at the $P = 0.05$ probability level.

Chapter 9

Regression and Correlation

Introduction

In Chapter 4 the everyday saying 'red sky at night, shepherds' delight' was mentioned. In effect this is a statement concerning an *association between two events*, namely the colour of the sky and the weather, albeit a very unscientific one. In a less trivial example, we might be considering the relationship between two quantities, X and Y, each of which can be measured on a scale. Two examples are: (*a*) dose and response, (*b*) habit and disease incidence, and the hypotheses investigated may be (*a*) whether an increase in a chemo-therapeutic drug dose produces a corresponding increase in tumour response, and (*b*) whether there is a correlation between smoking and lung cancer. If an association between X and Y is suspected, then the first step is to draw a *scatter diagram*, Figure 9.1, to give an indication of any possible *correlation* between X and Y. In the hypothetical example of Figure 9.1 it looks as if there is a *trend*, and that the points lie near a straight line.

Figure 9.1
Scatter diagram of points.
Is there a correlation between
X and Y?

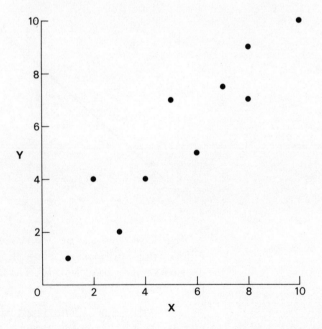

The topic of *correlation* is concerned with determining whether a *significant* association between X and Y *does* exist. Straight lines and curves which pass through the points on a scatter diagram and show a correlation are called *regression* lines and curves. The most common example is *linear regression* where the correlation is shown by a straight line on the scatter diagram.

A WORD OF WARNING!   The object of *proving* a correlation between X and Y is to show that a relationship exists between these two quantities, so that having demonstrated the existence of this relationship, it can be used within some theoretical framework.

However, *blind use* of regression formulae can be very misleading, for if Y = a *cause* and X = an *effect*, one must be careful not to draw too many conclusions if there may be several other possible causes. Cause and effect in medicine are seldom so simple as to be completely explained by a single straight line! The fact that a formula for a correlation coefficient, r, – see later – exists, which can be used for the data of Figure 9.2 and Figure 9.3, and quoted to seven decimal places, is no reason for saying that there is a linear relation between X and Y for Figures 9.2 and 9.3 data. It is the *size* of the correlation coefficient which is important in deciding if a relationship is linear. Also, remember always to use *absolute* values on scatter diagrams and *never* rates.

Figure 9.2
An example of when not to draw a regression line

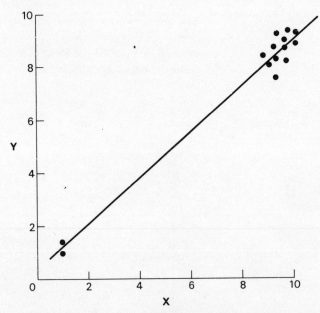

Even when there is an apparent *association* indicated by the scatter diagram, think twice before interpreting the association. The explanation must be meaningful. The flight of storks over Norway may be correlated to the birth rate *but* they still don't bring the babies!

The Equation of a Straight Line

Figure 9.4 is a graph on *linear* graph paper, with a vertical y-scale and a horizontal x-scale, of a straight line with an equation given in Formula 9.1.

Formula 9.1

$$y = ax + b$$

Figure 9.3
An example of when not to
draw a regression line

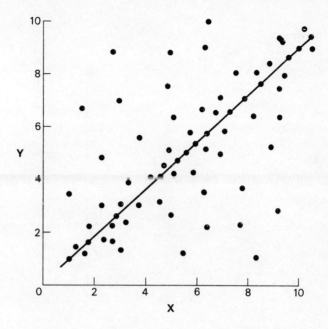

Eight points are marked on the *straight line* and these correspond to
x and *y* values given in Table 9.1. The (*x*, *y*) points are called *co-
ordinates*, (see page 5).

The points in the table can in fact be seen to have a pattern,
namely as *x* increases by 2, *y* also increases by 2, and they can all be
fitted by the equation

$$y = 1x - 2$$

which is of the same type as Formula 9.1 where a = 1 and b = −2.

Table 9.1
Co-ordinate points
of the straight line
in Figure 9.4

(x,	y)
(−4,	−6)
(−2,	−4)
(0,	−2)
(2,	0)
(4,	2)
(6,	4)
(8,	6)
(10,	8)

The quantity a is called the *slope* or *gradient* of the straight line,
and measures the rate at which it rises. In Figure 9.4, a = 1 which
implies that an increase in *x* produces the same increase in *y*. The
quantity b is called the *intercept* of the straight line, and is the
value of *y* where the straight line crosses the vertical *y*-axis. In this
example, b = − 2, and it is seen from Figure 9.4 that the line crosses
the *y*-axis when *y* = −2.

Figure 9.4
The equation of a straight
line

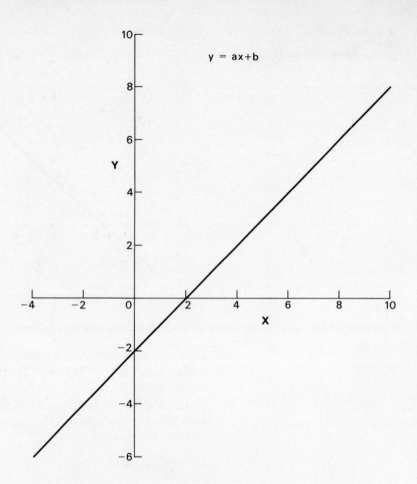

The Method of Least Squares

The example in Table 9.1 is an example in which *all* the eight points lie on a straight line. In practical problems, however, where the results are never as simple, a method is required to determine the a and b values of Formula 9.1. If six investigators draw the line by eye then there will probably be six different 'best fit' lines to the same data. To avoid this, several calculation methods are available, of which the most commonly used is the *method of least squares.* To illustrate the method, the data from Figure 9.1 will be used, see the first two columns of Table 9.2, which are headed x and y. The formulae required for calculating a and b are:

Formula 9.2
Intercept

$$\text{Intercept b} = \frac{\Sigma(x) \cdot \Sigma(xy) - \Sigma(x^2) \cdot \Sigma(y)}{[\Sigma(x)]^2 - N \cdot [\Sigma(x^2)]}$$

Formula 9.3
Slope

$$\text{Slope a} = \frac{\Sigma(x) \cdot \Sigma(y) - N \cdot [\Sigma(xy)]}{[\Sigma(x)]^2 - N \cdot [\Sigma(x^2)]}$$

N is the number of points on the scatter diagram, and for the example in Table 9.2, $N = 10$.

Table 9.2
Calculation of slope
a and intercept b by
the method of least
squares

x	y	x^2	xy
1	1	1	1
3	2	9	6
2	4	4	8
4	4	16	16
6	5	36	30
5	7	25	35
8	7	64	56
7	7.5	49	52.5
8	9	64	72
10	10	100	100

$\Sigma(x) = 54 \qquad \Sigma(y) = 56.5 \quad \Sigma(x^2) = 368 \quad \Sigma(xy) = 376.5$

$$a = \frac{\Sigma(x)\Sigma(y) - N[\Sigma(xy)]}{[\Sigma(x)]^2 - N[\Sigma(x^2)]}$$

$$= \frac{54 \times 56.5 - 10 \times 376.5}{(54)^2 - 10 \times 368}$$

$$= \frac{714}{764} = 0.93$$

$$b = \frac{\Sigma(x)\Sigma(xy) - \Sigma(x^2)\Sigma(y)}{[\Sigma(x)]^2 - N\Sigma(x^2)}$$

$$= \frac{54 \times 376.5 - 368 \times 56.5}{(54)^2 - 10 \times 368}$$

$$= \frac{461}{764} = 0.60$$

From these formulae it is seen that the four following summations are required: $\Sigma(x)$, $\Sigma(y)$, $\Sigma(xy)$, $\Sigma(x^2)$, where Σ means *sum of all the* ... *values.* From Table 9.2 the *least squares best fit straight line* is calculated:

$$y = (0.93)x + 0.60$$

and this has been drawn on the scatter diagram, Figure 9.1, and is seen in Figure 9.5. This straight line is called the *regression line of y on x* and may be used for predicting values of y for given values of x. This assumes that y is *dependent* upon x, and an example would be when y = tumour growth and x = time. Tumour growth can obviously be dependent on time; however, the reverse *cannot* be true, since time is *not* dependent upon tumour growth. Situations arise when it is not clear whether x depends on y or y depends on x. In that case, two regression lines are calculated y *on x* as in Figure 9.5 and also x *on y*. The choice of independent variable is then usually the one that will be used to predict values of the other. The regression equation can then be regarded as a prediction formula. If the correlation is good, then the two regression lines will be close together. The point at which they cross is $(\bar{x}, \bar{y})$ the sample mean, and this provides a good check on the arithmetic!

The method of least squares used to calculate the *best fit* straight line, minimises the squares of the deviations, (Δy) from the line. This is shown in Figure 9.5 where the vertical bars drawn from points to the line represent (Δy). The best fit straight line has been chosen such that the sum of all $(\Delta y)^2$ values is a minimum.

Figure 9.5
Regression line of y on x, showing the deviations Δy of the points from the line shown

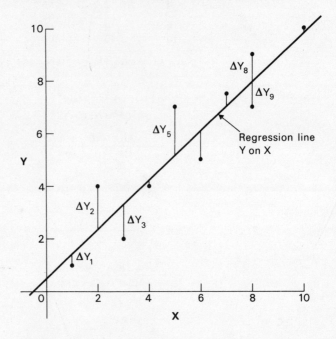

In Table 9.3 the *slope* a and the *intercept* b were calculated. The formulae for the standard errors in a and b are:

Formula 9.4
Standard error of slope

$$\sigma_a = \sqrt{\frac{N \cdot [\Sigma(\Delta y)^2]}{(N-2)\,[N\Sigma(x^2) - [\Sigma(x)]^2]}}$$

Formula 9.5
Standard error of intercept

$$\sigma_b = \sqrt{\frac{[\Sigma(\Delta y)^2] \cdot [\Sigma(x^2)]}{(N-2)\,[N\Sigma(x^2) - [\Sigma(x)]^2]}}$$

where $\Sigma(\Delta y)^2$ is the sum of the squares of the deviations of each point from the line.

Formula 9.6
Deviations Δy

$$(\Delta y) = \begin{bmatrix} y \text{ value of the} \\ \text{point on the} \\ \text{graph,} \\ observation \end{bmatrix} - \begin{bmatrix} (ax + b) \text{ which is} \\ \text{the } y\text{-value of the} \\ \text{point on the line} \\ calculated \text{ using} \\ \text{the straight line} \\ \text{formula} \end{bmatrix}$$

Using the formulae for σ_a and σ_b, and when quoting two standard errors, we have that a = 0.93 ± 0.28 and b = 0.60 ± 1.64.

Correlation Coefficient

The distribution of points scattered on the diagram Figure 9.1, makes it easy to visualise a linear relationship between y and x, with the straight line passing through the central section of the band of points. In statistical terminology, it can be said that *there is good correlation between y and x* and this can be shown numerically by calculating a *correlation coefficient* to describe the position of the straight line $y = ax + b$ relative to the observations. Formula 9.7 is the formula for the correlation coefficient r.

Formula 9.7
Coefficient, r

$$r = \frac{\Sigma[(x - \bar{x}) \cdot (y - \bar{y})]}{\sqrt{[\Sigma(x - \bar{x})^2] \cdot [\Sigma(y - \bar{y})^2]}}$$

An alternative, Formula 9.8, does not contain $\bar{x}$ and $\bar{y}$, but although it looks more complicated, many of the summation (Σ) terms have already been calculated to determine a and b in Table 9.3, and it is therefore more convenient to use in practice.

Formula 9.8
Coefficient, r

$$r = \frac{N[\Sigma(xy)] - [\Sigma(x) \cdot \Sigma(y)]}{\sqrt{[N[\Sigma(x^2)] - [\Sigma(x)]^2] \cdot [N[\Sigma(y^2)] - [\Sigma(y)]^2]}}$$

For a straight line such as that in Figure 9.5, we say that there is *positive correlation*, and this is indicated by the +ve sign for r, Figure 9.6.

Figure 9.6
Correlation

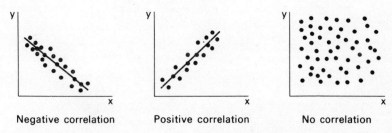

Negative correlation   Positive correlation   No correlation

Table 9.3 shows the calculation schedule for r using both Formula 9.7 and 9.8.

Testing for a Significant Correlation

In Table 9.3 it is seen that $r = +0.92$. A perfect positive correlation would be $r = +1$ and a perfect negative correlation would be $r = -1$. No correlation would be $r = 0$. A correlation coefficient of $r = +0.92$ is therefore good correlation.

r can be calculated for any scatter diagram using Formula 9.7 or 9.8. Whether the results show a *significant correlation* between x and y should then be tested before values of y are predicted using the straight line relationship. The significance test is made using the *t-test*, where the *t*-statistic is

Formula 9.9
t-statistic

$$t = \frac{r\sqrt{N-2}}{\sqrt{1-r^2}}$$

which is derived from $t = (r)/[\text{standard deviation of } r]$. The number of degrees of freedom is given by

Formula 9.10
Degrees of freedom

$$\nu = (N - 2)$$

where N is the number of points on the scatter diagram.

Table 9.3
Calculation schedule to determine a correlation coefficient

$$\Sigma x = 54, \bar{x} = 54/10 = 5.4$$
$$\Sigma y = 56.5, \bar{y} = 56.5/10 = 5.65$$

x	y	y^2 (used in method 2)	$x - \bar{x}$	$y - \bar{y}$	$(x - \bar{x})^2$	$(y - \bar{y})^2$	$(x - \bar{x})(y - \bar{y})$
1	1	1	−4.4	−4.65	19.36	21.62	20.46
3	2	4	−2.4	−3.65	5.76	13.32	8.76
2	4	16	−3.4	−1.65	11.56	2.72	5.61
4	4	16	−1.4	−1.65	1.96	2.72	2.31
6	5	25	0.6	−0.65	0.36	0.42	−0.39
5	7	49	−0.4	1.35	0.16	1.82	−0.54
8	7	49	2.6	1.35	6.76	1.82	3.51
7	7.5	56.25	1.6	1.85	2.56	3.42	2.96
8	9	81	2.6	3.35	6.76	11.22	8.71
10	10	100	4.6	4.35	21.16	18.92	20.01
		$\Sigma(y^2) = 397.25$			$\Sigma(x-\bar{x})^2$ $= 76.4$	$\Sigma(y-\bar{y})^2$ $= 78.0$	$\Sigma(x-\bar{x})(y-\bar{y})$ $= 71.4$

Method 1

$$r = \frac{\Sigma(x - \bar{x})(y - \bar{y})}{\sqrt{\Sigma(x - \bar{x})^2 \cdot \Sigma(y - \bar{y})^2}} \quad \text{from Formula 9.7}$$

$$= \frac{71.4}{\sqrt{(76.4 \times 78)}} = 0.92$$

Method 2

$$\Sigma x = 54$$
$$\Sigma y = 56.5$$
$$\Sigma xy = 376.5 \text{ from Table 9.2}$$
$$(\Sigma x)^2 = (54)^2 = 2916$$
$$(\Sigma y)^2 = (56.5)^2 = 3192.25$$
$$\Sigma x^2 = 368 \text{ from Table 9.2}$$
$$\Sigma y^2 = 397.25$$

$$r = \frac{N\Sigma xy - \Sigma x \Sigma y}{\sqrt{[N\Sigma x^2 - (\Sigma x)^2] \cdot [N\Sigma y^2 - (\Sigma y)^2]}} \quad \text{from Formula 9.8}$$

$$r = \frac{(10 \times 376.5) - (54 \times 56.5)}{\sqrt{[10 \times 368 - 2916] \cdot [10 \times 397.25 - 3192.25]}}$$

$$= \frac{714}{\sqrt{(764 \times 780.25)}}$$

$$= 0.92$$

The *null hypothesis, H_0,* is that *there is no linear associated between y and x*. Since $r = + 0.92$ and $N = 10$, from Formula 9.9,

$$t = \frac{0.92 \times 2.83}{\sqrt{1 - 0.846}} = + 6.6$$

Table 8.3 gives critical values of t for the t-test, for different degrees of freedom (ν) and for $P = 0.05$. When $\nu = (N - 2) = 8$, the critical value of t equals 2.31. The calculated t-statistic is 6.6, which is greater than 2.31, and we therefore *reject the null hypothesis, H_0,* and say that there is a significant correlation between x and y, at the $P = 0.05$ level.

The test we have just completed is a *two-tailed* test, $P = 2\alpha$ in the notation of Figure 6.2, since we have tested for a critical value of t greater than $+ 2.31$ or less than -2.31. If there is no linear association and H_0 is true, then the calculated t would have been greater than $+ 2.31$ or less than -2.31 in only 5 per cent of any series of identical trials with $N = 10$.

Figure 9.7
Data for 36 patients treated during 1945–1960 for T3NO glottic carcinoma, who died with disease present, males: aged 55–65 years

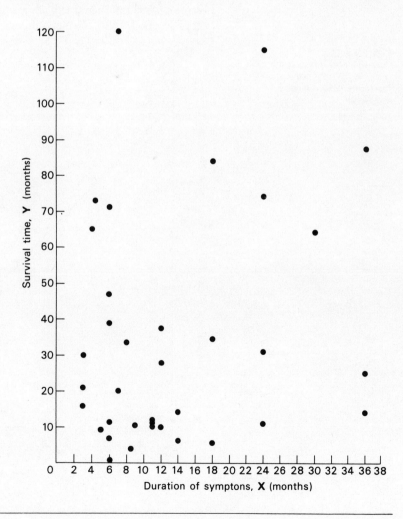

The preceding sections have inevitably been theoretical, with the necessary formulae explained using simple numbers unrelated to practical problems. The subsequent examples are included to demonstrate some of the practical problems where regression lines may — but in some cases should not — be drawn.

Figure 9.7 is a scatter diagram for the duration of symptoms prior to treatment of carcinoma larynx and the survival time subsequent to treatment, of cases eventually dying with their cancer present. From the diagram it is evident that there is *no correlation* between the two parameters, and that the shorter symptom durations are *not* related to the longer survival times. It *is* possible to draw a regression line and calculate a correlation coefficient using the methodology of Tables 9.2 and 9.3, by inserting the relevant numbers into the formulae. However, since there is obviously no correlation, it is meaningless to carry out the procedure.

Figure 9.8 shows the variation of annual death rates in England and Wales due to tuberculosis over the period 1900—1960. The points can be seen to lie approximately on a straight line, and a meaningful regression line can therefore be drawn to describe the trend over the 60 year period. Using the methodology of Tables 9.2 and 9.3, the regres-

Figure 9.8
Data for tuberculosis death rates per 100 000 population for 1900—1960, England and Wales

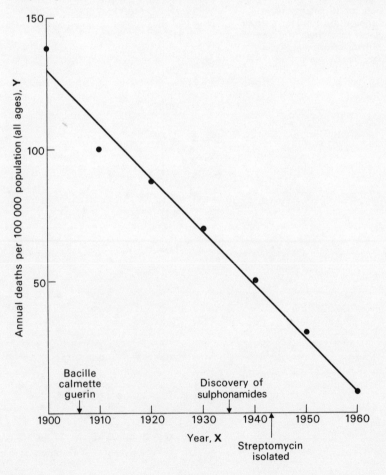

sion line is: $Y = -2X + 130$, and the correlation coefficient is $r = -0.99$, which is an example of very good *negative correlation*. In this example, the downward trend cannot continue indefinitely since it is already rapidly approaching zero. This illustrates the dangers of extrapolation of linear trends without due thought! The causes of the trend shown in Figure 9.8 are due to several factors including better public health and personal hygiene as the century progressed, the availability of immunisation using BCG and treatment using streptomycin.

Figure 9.10 is taken from the work of Doll and Hill on mortality in relation to smoking, and is an example of very good *positive correlation*, $r = +0.99$. However, it must be remembered that just because there is a good correlation between two variables X and Y this does not automatically prove that a certain cause and effect are directly related.

Figure 9.9 is another example of *positive correlation*, $r = +0.88$, which is not as good as that in Figure 9.10. Indeed, it is seen from the diagram that, after 1958 there is a marked periodicity in the pattern of deaths, with minima in 1962 and 1968. Although there is an upward trend in the death rate, the correlation is not good enough to predict the rate for years subsequent to 1972.

Figure 9.9
Data for crude death rates in England and Wales, 1946–1972, per million population, due to motor vehicle traffic accidents

Figure 9.10
Data for annual death rates due to lung cancer, standardised for age; after Doll and Hill (1964) *British Medical Journal,* **1,** 1402.

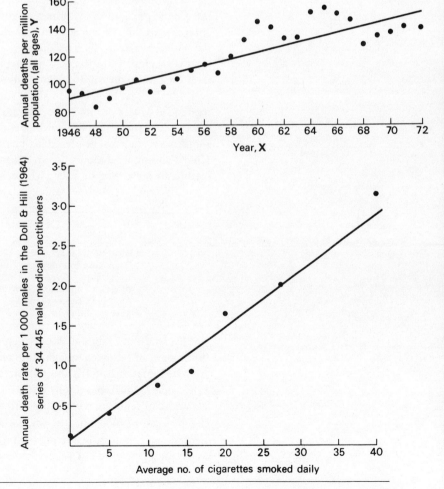

Chapter 10

Calculation of Survival Rates

Introduction

The title of this chapter includes the words *survival rates* but it could equally well have been *survival fractions* or *survival probabilities* since all three terms are linked. 50 per cent T-year survival *rate* is equivalent to a 0.50 T-year survival *fraction*, and a *probability* of survival of 1 chance in 2. What *is important* is a clear understanding of the conditions under which the survival is stated. For example, (*a*) whether it refers only to a single cause of death; (*b*) whether there has been an *adjustment* for cases lost to follow-up; (*c*) whether a comparison for a treated group has been made with a similar group by age and sex of the general population. Without a clearly defined rate, meaningful comparisons cannot be made between different sets of results even though they refer to the same disease.

It is also important to know the *method* of calculation of survival rates used by an investigator, since this will indicate how much of the available data has been used to assess survival. If series of patients treated for cancer or some other chronic disease whose progress is assessed by survival, are followed-up annually on their treatment anniversary, they can be placed in one of the five groups in Table 10.1 at any time subsequent to treatment. An example of a good method of presenting such data has been shown in Figure 1.2 using a *dot diagram*.

Table 10.1

Patient follow-up groups

GROUP	PATIENT FOLLOW-UP
1	Dead from cancer
2	Dead from an intercurrent disease, i.e. not cancer
3	Alive with no sign of recurrence
4	Alive with cancer present
5	Lost to follow-up

There are three methods for calculating a T-year survival rate, and the amount of follow-up information required for each method is given in Table 10.2. If T is short term, then it is not necessary to use a prediction model, but if long term, then a model will have the advantage of reducing the waiting period before a result can be given. The life table method will also produce a result earlier than the direct method, but not as early as a prediction model. However, satisfactory prediction models are not yet available for all cancer sites.

Table 10.2
Methods of calculating
survival rates

Method of Calculation	Basic data required for T-year rate	Applications
1. *Direct*	All cases observed to T	General
2. *Life Table*	At least some cases observed to T	General
3. *Prediction Model* (For use with long term survival tates only)	It is not necessary for any cases to have been observed to T	Cancer only

The Direct Method

To calculate the T-year survival rate by the direct method, the ratio in Formula 10.1 is computed.

Formula 10.1
T-year survival
rate

$$\text{T-year Survival Rate} = \frac{(\text{No. surviving at least T years})}{\begin{array}{l}(\text{No. entering for treatment at} \\ \text{time } T = 0 \text{ excluding those lost} \\ \text{to follow-up before } T)\end{array}}$$

The Life Table Method

In the direct method, the incomplete information relevant to cases lost to follow-up before time T has to be ignored completely when calculating the survival rate. The advantage of the life table method is that the incomplete follow-up information is not discarded.

To illustrate the life table method, the data in Table 10.3 and the notation in Table 10.4 will be used.

Table 10.3
Survival history of
150 patients treated
for cancer on
January 1st 1960

Year (From Jan. 1st — Dec. 31st)	Interval No. = i	Number dying during the interval = d_i		Number lost to follow-up during the interval = w_i
		From cancer = d_i^{CA}	From intercurrent disease = d_i^{ID}	
1960	1	38	1	4
1961	2	18	1	2
1962	3	12	0	1
1963	4	6	0	1
1964	5	4	2	0
1965	6	3	2	1
1966	7	2	1	2
1967	8	0	1	1
1968	9	0	3	4
1969	10	1	1	4

No. alive on Jan. 1st 1970 = 34

The total cases l_i entering the first interval ($i = 1$) will be all the cases treated on January 1st 1960, $l_1 = 150$. Further values of l_i that is l_2, $l_3, l_4, \ldots l_{10}$, will be calculated by subtracting the $(d_i + w_i)$ values in an 'ith' interval from the total cases, l_i, entering that interval,

Table 10.4
Notation for life
table method
referring to
cancer

Symbol	Definition
i	Interval number, see Table 10.3
d_i	*Total deaths* (cancer and intercurrent disease) in interval i
w_i	Total cases lost to follow-up in interval i
l_i	Total cases entering the ith interval
n_i	Number exposed to the risk of dying in the ith interval
q_i	Probability of dying *in* the ith interval
P_i	Probability of surviving *to* the end of the ith interval

Formula 10.2. Those patients who have 'dropped out' of an interval by death or loss, can no longer enter future intervals.

$$l_{i+1} = (l_i) - (d_i + w_i)$$

The calculations of l_i values for the data of Table 10.3 using Formula 10.2 are given in Table 10.5 and it can be seen that the last figure of $l_{11} = 34$ agrees with the value, 34, on the last line of Table 10.3.

Table 10.5

Calculations using
Formula 10.2

```
        No. entering at T = 0 is l₁  = 150
                        thus l₂  = 150 − (38 + 1 + 4) = 107
                             l₃  = 107 − (18 + 1 + 2) =  86
                             l₄  =  86 − (12 + 0 + 1) =  73
                             l₅  =  73 − (6  + 0 + 1) =  66
                             l₆  =  66 − (4  + 2 + 0) =  60
                             l₇  =  60 − (3  + 2 + 1) =  54
                             l₈  =  54 − (2  + 1 + 2) =  49
                             l₉  =  49 − (0  + 1 + 1) =  47
                             l₁₀ =  47 − (0  + 3 + 4) =  40
        and no. entering the
        11th interval on Jan.
        1st 1970 is          l₁₁ =  40 − (1  + 1 + 4) =  34
```

We must now return to *probabilities*, since the life table survival rates are calculated by multiplying together a series of probabilities — see Law 2 of mathematical probability, page 20. The probability of dying in the ith interval denoted by q_i, Table 10.4, is the ratio, given in Formula 10.3.

$$q_i = \frac{(\text{No. of deaths in the interval})}{\left[\begin{array}{c} \text{No. exposed to the risk} \\ \text{of dying during the interval} \end{array}\right]} = d_i/n_i$$

The number exposed to the risk of dying in the ith interval, n_i, requires a little more amplification. In contrast to the direct method, the life table method assumes that: *the patients lost to follow-up during the ith interval were exposed to the risk of dying, on average, for half the interval.* This is the basic assumption of the life table method which enables the data on the *lost to follow-up* cases to be utilised. Using this assumption, we have that

Formula 10.4
No. exposed to
risk of dying

$$n_i = [\text{Total cases entering the } i^{\text{th}} \text{ interval}, l_i] - \tfrac{1}{2} \cdot w_i$$

and therefore from Formula 10.3

$$q_i = \frac{d_i}{(l_i - \tfrac{1}{2}w_i)}$$

which is the probability of dying *in* a given i^{th} interval. Since the total probability is 1, $(1 - q)$ is the probability of surviving *in* the interval. The words *in* and *to* are most important in this context.

The probability of surviving *to* a given year T subsequent to treatment, implies that survival has been achieved throughout *all* the ith intervals prior to year T. The probability of survival to T is therefore given by the product of individual annual survival probabilities, and is calculated using Formula 10.6,

$$P_T = (1 - q_1) \cdot (1 - q_2) \cdot (1 - q_3) \ldots (1 - q_i)$$

where year T is the end point of the ith interval, Table 10.3.

The arithmetic required for Formula 10.6 for T-year rates between 1 and 10 years is shown in Table 10.6. This method gives 0.52 for the 3-year survival rate, compared with a value of $\frac{(80 - 7)}{(150 - 7)} = 0.51$ using the direct method. However, greater discrepancies between the two methods occur for longer term survival rates. For the 10-year rate, the direct method gives $\frac{(54 - 20)}{(150 - 20)} = 0.26$ whereas the life table method gives 0.32. Ideal series of data will have complete follow-up, but in practice this is hardly ever achieved, and the life table method which takes into account *all available information* will give a better estimate of the long term survival rates than the direct method.

In the example illustrated, the T-year survival rate has been calculated for *all* causes of death, cancer *and* intercurrent. It is however possible to modify the schedule to calculate the T-year survival rate for a specific cause of death, say cancer. In this instance the calculations in Table 10.5 would be modified such that:

1. Column d_i becomes d_i^{CA} and refers to cancer deaths only.

2. Column w_i becomes $(w_i + d_i^{ID})$ and refers to cases lost to follow-up *plus* intercurrent deaths.

3. Column n_i becomes $(l_i - \tfrac{1}{2}w_i - \tfrac{1}{2}d_i^{ID})$ since those dying from intercurrent disease can also be assumed to be exposed to the risk of dying from cancer, on average, for half the interval.

The procedure is then as before.

Table 10.6
Life table calculation (from: Mould, 1976, Clinical Radiology, Vol. 27, p. 33)

Interval end point Year T Dec. 31st	Interval number i	Deaths d_i From Table 10.3	Losses w_i From Table 10.3	Total entering l_i See Table 10.5	No. at risk $n_i = (l_i - \frac{1}{2}w_i)$	Prob. of dying in interval i $q_i = d_i/n_i$	Prob. of surviving in interval i $(1-q_i)$	Probability of surviving to year T (The T-year SURVIVAL RATE) $P_T = (1-q_1)\ldots(1-q_i)$
1960	1	39	4	150	148	0.263	0.737	0.737
1961	2	19	2	107	106	0.179	0.821	0.605
1962	3	12	1	86	85.5	0.140	0.860	0.520
1963	4	6	1	73	72.5	0.082	0.918	0.477
1964	5	6	0	66	66	0.090	0.910	0.434
1965	6	5	1	60	59.5	0.084	0.916	0.397
1966	7	3	2	54	53	0.056	0.944	0.374
1967	8	1	1	49	48.5	0.020	0.980	0.366
1968	9	3	4	47	45	0.066	0.934	0.341
1969	10	2	4	40	38	0.052	0.948	0.323
1970	11			34				

It must also be pointed out that most series requiring analysis will not have had *all* patients treated on the same day, such as January 1st 1960 as in Table 10.3, but would have different dates within a specified treatment interval. The life table method is just as relevant for this situation though, and the only alterations required to Tables 10.3 and 10.6 are the removal of the first column, which was quoted for convenience and is not essential for the calculations. The patient data is placed within relevant annual intervals.

LIFE TABLES FOR A GENERAL POPULATION   Table 10.6 is a life table, but it is relevant only to a specially selected group of people, and not to the general population of England and Wales. Life tables which are relevant to the general population are published at regular intervals by the Registrar General, and Table 10.7 is an extract from one such table.

Table 10.7
English Life Table,
No. 12, Males

Age x	l_x	d_x	p_x	q_x	$\overset{o}{e}_x$
0	100,000	2449	0.97551	0.02449	68.09
1	97,551	153	0.99843	0.00157	68.80
2	97,398	96	0.99901	0.00099	67.80
3	97,302	67	0.99931	0.00069	66.97
4	97,235	..	..	..	..

For this table, an anniversary date is a *birth date* rather than a *treatment date*, there are no losses to follow-up and an additional quantity, $\overset{o}{e}_x$ is also tabulated. The life table is a particular way of expressing *death rates* experienced by a given population.

For an explanation of Table 10.7, let us imagine *100 000 infants*, all born on the same day and dying as they passed through each year of life at the same rate as was experienced at each of these ages by the population of England and Wales in 1960–1962. Now refer to Table 10.8.

Table 10.8
Life table notation

Symbol	Definition
x	*Age*
l_x	*Number of infants alive* at each birth anniversary.
d_x	*Number dying* in a given year. (Thus if 2449 died in the first year, i.e. between $x = 0$ and $x = 1$, then l_x for the row $x = 1$ will be: $100000 - 2449 = 97551$).
p_x	The *probability of living* from age x to age $(x + 1)$.
q_x	The *probability of dying* in the year defined by the limits x and $(x + 1)$. (Thus $[p + q_x] = 1$, since individuals must either live or die in a given year).
$\overset{o}{e}_x$	The *life expectation*, or average length of life.

There is also another important quantity m_x which is the death rate at age x last birth anniversary.

Formula 10.7
Death rate

$$m_x = \frac{\text{Average deaths at age } x \text{ last anniversary}}{\text{Average population at age } x \text{ last anniversary}}$$

m_x refers to an average population, and the mid-period (if we are dealing in annual rates, then it is the mid-year) population is used as an approximation. The mid-year population will be $(l_x - \frac{1}{2}d_x)$, assuming that the death rate is uniform throughout the year, $\frac{1}{2}$ of the d_x deaths will occur before mid-year and $\frac{1}{2}$ of the d_x deaths will occur after mid-year. Formula 10.7 thus becomes:

Formula 10.8
Death rate

$$m_x = \frac{d_x}{(l_x - \frac{1}{2}d_x)}$$

The probabilities p_x and q_x may be calculated from a knowledge of m_x as follows, using the fact that $q_x = (d_x/l_x)$ and $p_x + q_x = 1$.

Formula 10.9
Probability of
dying (q_x)

$$q_x = \left[\frac{2m_x}{2 + m_x}\right] = \left[\frac{m_x}{1 + \frac{1}{2}m_x}\right] \text{ and } p_x = \left[\frac{2 - m_x}{2 + m_x}\right]$$

The Prediction Model Method

When a large number of patients are treated for cancer, it is reasonable to assume that a proportion, C, will be permanently cured. The remaining fraction, $(1 - C)$, will be liable to die of cancer if they do not previously die of an intercurrent disease. If an assumption can be made for a formula to describe the distribution curve of survival times of cases who die with cancer present which is the $(1 - C)$ group, then a statistical model can be constructed (see Figures 3.4 and 3.5). The variable parameters of the model will be the shape constants of the assumed distribution curve and the proportion C.

Figure 10.1 is a schematic diagram of a model for carcinoma cervix with a positively skewed theoretical curve for the distribution of survival times. The T-year survival rate, when *only cancer deaths are considered*, is given by Formula 10.10.

Figure 10.1
Prediction model

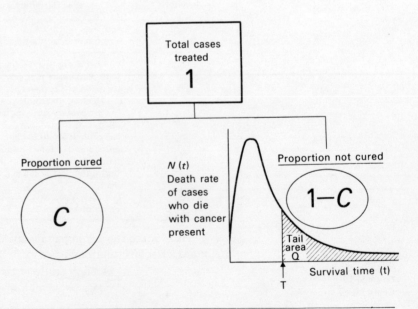

Total cases treated
1

Proportion cured

C

$N(t)$
Death rate of cases who die with cancer present

Proportion not cured

$1-C$

Tail area Q

Survival time (t)

T

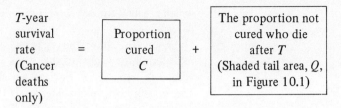

| T-year survival rate (Cancer deaths only) | = | Proportion cured C | + | The proportion not cured who die after T (Shaded tail area, Q, in Figure 10.1) |

Formula 10.10

T-year survival rate (Cancer deaths only) $= C + (1 - C) \cdot Q$

For a further discussion of a prediction model of the type in Figure 10.1 see Mould and Boag (1975) *British Journal of Cancer*, Vol. 32, 529–550, where it has been shown that a prediction model can provide a useful alternative to the life table method of calculating survival rates, even when follow-up data is sufficiently extensive to allow the latter method to be used. The method certainly extracts more information from the clinical data than does the crude direct method of calculation, and it offers the unique advantage that an early prediction of longer term results can be made, within calculable error limits.

The Concept of Cure in Cancer

Survival to 5-years subsequent to treatment has often been regarded as a criterion indicative of a *cure* from cancer. Although it may be convenient and simple to use, it is not always a good representation of the measure of success for all forms of cancer. It can, however, be counted as satisfactory for those cancers where recurrence after treatment is usually rapid, since it will then give considerable hope of permanent cure. The equating of *cure* with a general *T-year survival rate* is, therefore, only logical when values of T are specified for individual cancers. Survival results may depend to a variable degree on factors such as clinical stage of the disease at diagnosis, histological type of growth and type of treatment.

The distribution of ages of a group of patients treated for cancer is important since the life expectancy of those in the first two or three decades of life is greater than for those in their seventies. Allowance should be made for this age factor when interpreting survival results in cancer.

If as a trivial example we assume that 100 patients were treated for one particular cancer, and that they were all age 85 years on treatment, one would hardly expect a high 10-year survival rate, since the life expectancy of males within the general population who have reached the age of 85 years is only some 3.5 years. A more efficient measure of success than the crude T-year survival rate, would thus be the ratio:

Formula 10.11
Age corrected
survival rate

$$100 \times \left[\frac{\text{(crude T-year survival rate)}}{\begin{array}{c} \text{(expected T-year survival rate in the normal} \\ \text{population for a group of people with the} \\ \text{same age distribution as the treated group)} \end{array}} \right] \%$$

which is called the *age corrected* T-year survival rate, expressed as a percentage.

Figure 10.2 shows the crude and corrected 5- to 15-year survival rates for all the cancer of the cervix and cancer of the tongue patients who were registered in England and Wales in 1954—55, and for whom a 15-year follow-up is now known. If the patients were all relatively young at treatment, the expected T-year survival rate in the normal population would be high and the crude and age corrected T-year survival rates would be similar. It is seen in Figure 10.2 that for the cancers shown, there is a large difference between crude and age corrected rates, and this emphasises the need to be aware of exactly which type of rate is quoted when comparing survival results from different publications.

Figure 10.2
Crude and age corrected survival rates. Registrar General's data for 1954—1955 registrations, England and Wales

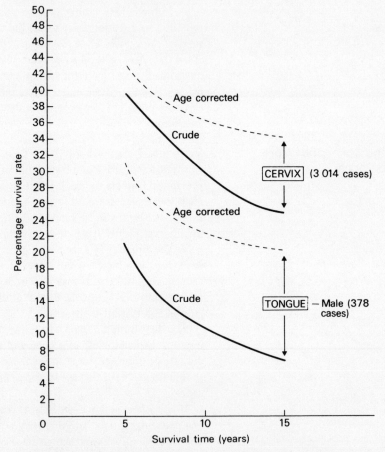

The value of the year T at which a permanent cure might be considered to have occurred for a group of patients by cancer site, age, treatment, . . . etc., has been suggested as that time after treatment when the *annual death rate from all causes* is similar to that of a *normal population group* of the same sex and age distribution. An estimate of the year T can be made graphically as in Figure 10.3 by a comparison of observed and expected survival curves, and such a

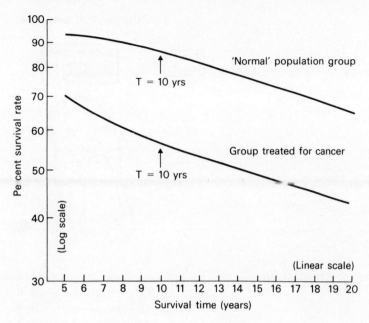

Figure 10.3
Demonstration of a concept
for cure in patients treated
for cancer, data for 337
stage 1 carcinoma cervix
patients treated 1944—1954

study has been undertaken for patients treated 1932—1949 at the
Christie Hospital, Manchester, Easson and Russell (1968) *The Curability
of Cancer in Various Sites*, Pitman.

When using this concept of cure for those sites where it can be
demonstrated, the critical year is often about the 10th after treatment
when the two curves become parallel. An example of an earlier T is testis
cancer and an example of a cancer in which very late recurrences are
prone to occur and this concept of cure cannot be demonstrated, is
cancer of the breast. That is not to say, however, that there are no permanent cures for cancer of the breast, but only that a death rate from
all causes similar to that of the general population cannot be demonstrated even 15 years after treatment.

Earlier it was theorised that there does in fact exist a proportion
of patients who are *permanently cured* following treatment for cancer
and this was denoted by the letter *C* in Figure 10.1. Estimates of *C*
obtained using prediction model methods are shown in Table 10.9.

Table 10.9
Estimates of C for carcinoma
cervix patients treated at
four London teaching
hospitals, 1944—1962

Disease stage at diagnosis	Total number of cases	$C \pm 1$ Standard Error
1	744	0.62 ± 0.02
2	1 327	0.40 ± 0.01
3	758	0.20 ± 0.02

Cancer Registration and Survival Follow-up in England and Wales

Efficient cancer registration, survival follow-up, data storage and data
retrieval are essential for any analysis of survival results for patients
treated over a period of years, but it must be remembered that a com-
puter will not automatically solve all the problems. The *Ostrich Syn-
drome* is to be avoided!

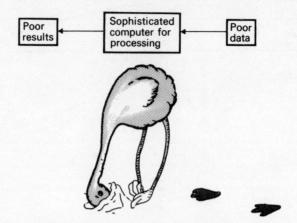

Hospital Registration

No single method of recording and updating cancer case histories has been adopted by British hospitals. For convenience in storage and retrieval, some have transferred their pre-1944 records to microfilm, but most of the information is still to be found in typed and hand-written notes. Usually, both the original case history and a summary system are available. The latter can take the form of entries in specially printed books, or on a series of ordinary filing cards. Individual filing systems differ and records can be arranged in order of treatment year or patient hospital number, or subdivided into dead or alive groups.

Finally, it is important to remember that together with efficient follow-up records subsequent to treatment, full *up-to-date* charted records must be kept during treatment. These can provide a very useful basis when planning prospective clinical trials, and are of immense help in providing guidance on the management of the rarer diseases.

Regional Registration

There are fourteen *regional* cancer registries in England and Wales, Figure 10.4, and the *hospital* cancer registries in each region send data on all their patients to the regional registries. The data is entered on record cards provided by the region, but does not include all the information in Table 10.10 which is probably the minimum required for any useful retrospective *survival* study on cancer treatment. For example, since 1970, item 6, *clinical disease stage at diagnosis* is no longer recorded even for sites such as breast and cervix, and one only has to refer to Table 10.9 to see the influence of disease stage on survival. However, it must be remarked that Regional Cancer Registries provide a very useful function as data banks for epidemiological studies, when survival after treatment is not the parameter of interest, and the investigations are concerned more with factors affecting the incidence of a disease, (e.g. occupation, age).

National Registration

The regional registries submit data on a voluntary basis to the National Registry, which is a part of the Office of Population Censuses and

Surveys (OPCS) under the Registrar General's aegis. Because of the multitude of people and organisations involved in transmitting data, the inevitable room for error can be imagined and it is therefore not difficult to see why only broadly based statistics are produced at regional and national level. It is also relevant to record that the OPCS now no longer expect the Regional Registries to provide them with *any* survival follow-up data on patients registered after January 1st 1976. The OPCS will in future obtain notification of the death of a cancer patient from the National Health Service Central Register (which contains all persons

Table 10.10
Patient Data
Parameters

1	Date of first treatment
2	Date of recurrence (if any)
3	Date of death
	i) Cause of death
	ii) Post mortem?
4	Patient state (dead or alive) at yearly anniversaries subsequent to the date of the first treatment
5	Details of treatment
6	Clinical disease stage at diagnosis
7	Tumour histology
8	Age at diagnosis
9	Sex
10	Hospital centre at which first treatment was given.

Figure 10.4
Regional cancer registries in
England and Wales, boundaries
before April 1st 1974

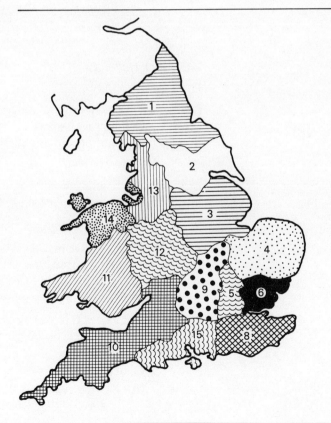

with an NHS number) but this will only provide the date of death and not the cause.

SUMMARY   From the foregoing discussion, it is apparent that it is usually practical to store detailed case history information such as that in Table 10.10 only at a *hospital* level, since *all* cases are required, not a random selection, and parameters such as method of treatment and definition of clinical stage sub-divisions can vary between hospitals. If the hospital registry cannot provide adequate information then there is no alternative to a *do-it-yourself* method of abstracting the data from the individual case notes.

Glossary of Incidence, Prevalence, Survival and Death Rate Terminology

AGE SPECIFIC RATES   Refer to the rates for specific age groups for each sex. The definition of the age groups will depend on the nature of the disease and its distribution in the population. However, it is wise to ensure that the age groups fall into one or more of the five year age intervals used by the Registrar General in official publications on population.

AGE CORRECTED RATES   See above, *Age Specific Rates*, and Formula 10.11 for the age corrected *survival* rate.

ANNUAL PREVALENCE RATE

$$\frac{\text{(No. of specified persons manifesting a disease in a stated year)}}{\text{(Average No. of such persons at risk during that year)}} \times 1\ 000$$

CASE FATALITY RATE   The death rate amongst those known to have a specific disease.

CRUDE RATE   Refers to the average rate for the whole population. Unless populations have a similar age structure and similar sex structure, the crude rate can be misleading when making comparisons. See *Age Specific Rates*.

CURE RATE   This is a measure of *new* cases of a disease, and is usually expressed as a proportion per 1 000 population at risk. An annual incidence will be:

CURE INDEX 'C'   Used in conjunction with statistical models for predicting long-term survival rates following treatment for cancer, see Figure 10.1. *C* may be thought of as the survival rate at infinite time, when causes of death other than cancer are ignored.

INCIDENCE RATE   This is a measure of *new* cases of a disease and is usually expressed as a proportion per 1000 population at risk. An annual incidence will be:

$$\frac{\text{(No. of new cases of a disease in one year)}}{\text{(Average no. of persons at risk in that group during that year)}} \times 1\ 000$$

INFANT MORTALITY   The number of deaths of infants in the *first year* of life stated per 1 000 live births.

MORTALITY   The death rate or mortality is the proportion of persons dying from a disease or set of diseases (i.e. a *cause* or *multiple causes* or *all causes*). The rate might be expressed per 1 000, 10 000, 100 000 or per million population at risk.

NEONATAL MORTALITY   Deaths of infants in the *first four weeks* of life stated per 1 000 live births.

PERINATAL MORTALITY   Number of stillbirths *plus* the number of deaths in the first week of life stated per 1 000 total live *and* still-births.

POINT PREVALENCE RATE

$$\frac{\text{(No. of specified persons manifesting a disease at any one time)}}{\text{(No. of persons at risk)}} \times 1\ 000$$

PREVALENCE RATE   Refers to *all* cases and not only to new cases. The prevalence of a disease is determined by its incidence *and* duration. The incidence of carcinoma-in-situ of the cervix is thought to be extremely low but as the condition may continue to be in-situ for many years, the prevalence rate will be much higher than the incidence rate. Prevalence of a disease is usually measured either as a *Point Prevalence Rate* or as an *Annual Prevalence Rate*.

STANDARD POPULATION   See *Standardised Rate.*

STANDARDISED MORTALITY RATIO   Is a comparison of actual deaths in a particular population compared with those which would be expected in the *standard* population.

STANDARDISED RATE   Is a rate which has been compounded to take into account differences in the age and sex structure of the population over several areas and is therefore considered to refer to an *average* or *standard* population.

STILL BIRTH RATE   Number of still births expressed per 1 000 total live *and* still births.

SURVIVAL FRACTION   A T-year survival fraction is the proportion of persons surviving to T-years, stated as a number between 0 and 1.

SURVIVAL RATE   Proportion of persons surviving to T-years, stated either as a percentage between 0 and 100 per cent or as a number between 0 and 1, see *Survival Fraction*, and *Cure Index C.*

Chapter 11

Clinical Trials

Introduction

The results of a clinical trial in oncology will often be assessed by using a long term T-year survival rate as a criterion of success. An alternative is a sequential type of trial which is appropriate when the result can be assessed in the short term, for example local tumour regression at six months subsequent to treatment. Sequential trials are also relevant in medical fields other than oncology, when patients can be *paired* and a preference recorded for one of the two patients. The clinical assessment will be made without knowledge of the allocation to treatment A or B of each patient in the pair. This is termed a *blind* trial, and is designed to eliminate any bias on the part of the clinical assessor.

Only these two types of trial will be discussed in this chapter and for further reading, Armitage (1975) *Sequential Medical Trials*, Blackwell; and Harris and Fitzgerald (1970) *The Principles and Practice of Clinical Trials*, Livingstone, are recommended.

Decision Making Prior
to the Start of a Trial

Before beginning a clinical trial, several decisions *must* be taken, and seven general considerations are listed below:

1. The *population* taking part in the trial must be defined. In a trial in oncology this will involve defining the disease stage, site, sex, histology and catchment area. For a sequential trial where patients have to be paired, care must be taken not to define the matching characteristics so *narrowly* that too few pairs could be expected to be obtained to complete the trial in a reasonable time, *or so broadly* that the final results are of little value. It will often be found that co-ordination among several treatment centres will be necessary to obtain the required patient numbers. Additional care will then have to be taken to ensure uniformity between centres in the administration of the trial protocol.
2. The *treatment method* must be clearly defined, and the schedule must *not* be altered during the course of the trial.
3. The *criterion of success* must be accurately defined. For the first type of trial mentioned this will be a T-year survival rate, or a proportion cured, C, Figure 10.1. For the sequential trial, the criterion may be less objective and be stated in terms of complete regression (CR), partial regression (PR) and no change (NC).
4. It is also necessary to define by *what method the criteria are to be measured*. For T-year survival rates, this has been discussed in the preceding chapter. For the more subjective type of criteria, it must be ensured that the method is unequivocal.

5. The *length of time* the trial is going to last will be related to the patient intake. For the T-year survival rate trial this can be fixed approximately, given the patient intake and α- and β-risks. For the sequential trial there will be a built-in *stopping rule* in the trial design, although the trial length can be estimated in terms of a range of *number of patient pairs.*
6. Acceptable values for the α-risk and β-risk critical probability levels must be fixed, and will depend upon the consequences following errors in a final analysis in the trial. They will not be determined by convention alone and always set at $P_\alpha = 0.05$.
7. A decision must be made on *what improvement in the criterion of success would be considered worthwhile.* This will be related to the α- and β-risks and the total number of patients required for the trial.

Randomisation

In a clinical trial it is important that there is no *bias* which will make the results invalid. It is therefore necessary to allot patients into trial's treatment groups, A and B, by a method which eliminates any preconceived opinions that a particular patient might be more suitable for A than B. In other words, the intake into the two treatment groups must be *randomised.*

How NOT to randomise!
(*Courtesy: Evening Standard*)

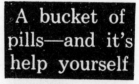

A bucket of pills—and it's help yourself

THE DOCTOR who piled all the drugs in his surgery into a bucket in the waiting room attaching a label telling his patients to help themselves and not bother him;

Even when the GMC did act it could get the oddest answers—the doctor with the pills in the plastic bucket simply retorted that his treatment was no more random than other doctors.

SINGLE RANDOMISATION Methods of randomisation are varied, some depend on birth dates (this is an approximation since the number of odd dates does not equal the number of even dates) and others on tables of random numbers. Using tables, the method is to allot one treatment for an odd number and the second treatment for an even number. This is *single randomisation.* Table 11.1 is the first row of random numbers taken from p. 12 of Lindley and Miller: *Cambridge Elementary Statistical Tables, 1968.*

Table 11.1
Random numbers

20 17 42 28 23 17 59 66 38 61 02 10 86 10 51 55 92 52 44 25

There are twenty pairs of two-digit numbers. If Treatment A = Odd Number and Treatment B = Even Number, and we have twenty patients entering the trial, then patients would be allocated for treatment as in Table 11.2.

BALANCED RANDOMISATION   From this table, however, it is seen that there are 8 treatment As and 12 treatment Bs, that is, an unequal final division between the two treatment groups. If the approximate number of patients who will enter the trial is known, then it is possible to have *balanced randomisation*, in which a certain block number of patients, say 50, will be balanced 25 for A and 25 for B. For the patients in Table 11.2, balanced randomisation would occur if the 18th and 19th patients were re-allocated to treatment A, thus making an equal number of patients for treatments A and B.

Table 11.2
Single randomisation

Patient	Treatment	Patient	Treatment
1	B	11	B
2	A	12	B
3	B	13	B
4	B	14	B
5	A	15	A
6	A	16	A
7	A	17	B
8	B	18	B
9	B	19	B
10	A	20	A

STRATIFIED RANDOMISATION   Another type of randomisation is *stratified randomisation* Figure 11.1, when the intake consists of two distinct classes, X and Y, for example, male and female, and the aim is to ensure that no matter how many of the intake are in class X or Y, half in each class receive treatment A and half receive treatment B. A balancing process must also be made in this situation.

Figure 11.1
Stratified randomisation

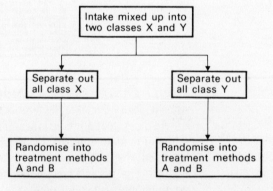

Number of Patients Required for a Cancer Trial with Proportion Cured as a Criterion

It has already been mentioned that *α-risk*, *β-risk* and *number of patients* required for a trial are all inter-related. Let us further assume that the *criterion of success* in this particular trial is going to be either the *proportion cured, C,* Figure 10.1 or a *long-term T-year survival rate*, such as the 10-year or 15-year rate. If the criterion of success is denoted by C_1 and C_2 for the two groups, then the *null hypothesis, H_0,* to be tested is $C_1 = C_2$.

The α-risk acceptable for the null hypothesis H_0 is usually set at $\alpha = 0.05$, although trials have been reported where the α-risk chosen was 0.01 or 0.10. If a significant result is obtained, H_0 is *rejected* and the logical course of action is to discontinue the worse treatment and concentrate on that one which has been shown to be significantly better. It is therefore important not to set too high a value for α, in order to avoid accepting one type of treatment as better than another, when a longer trial with a larger patient intake might have revealed no difference between them. There may of course be important differences in the side effects of the two treatments and in the absence of any significant difference between the primary criteria of success, that is, if H_0 is *accepted*, these side effects may properly become the determining factor in the choice of treatment.

If we have an alternative hypothesis H_1, then the β-risk is the risk of accepting the null hypothesis H_0 when the alternative hypothesis H_1 is true. When the χ^2 statistic is used to test for the significance of any difference between two T-year long term survival rates, or two proportions cured C_A and C_B, using a 2 x 2 contingency table, (Chapter 7), the quantity $(1 - \beta)$, called the *power of the test*, is defined as *the chance of getting a conclusive result in a single trial.*

Very few authors who have published results of cancer treatment have considered the β-risk although it is of particular interest when assessing the size of a clinical trial designed to give a significant result. However, to plan a single trial which will have a reasonably high chance, $(1 - \beta) = 0.90$, of giving a significant answer when differences between C_A and C_B of some 10 per cent are all that can be expected, needs very many patients as can be seen from Table 11.3, and such a trial could only be conducted in a reasonable time by co-operation between several centres.

Table 11.3
Number of patients required for a clinical trial, as a function of the α-risk ($P = 0.05$), the β-risk ($1 - \beta = 0.5$ or 0.75), and the observed difference in C values

Observed difference, $(C_A - C_B)$, which should be statistically significant at the $P = 0.05$ (α-risk) level	Total number of cases required for the clinical trial = $2N$ (N in group A and N in group B)	
	$(1 - \beta) = 0.5$ — A *1 in 2 chance* of getting a conclusive result in a single trial	$(1 - \beta) = 0.75$ — A *3 in 4 chance* of getting a conclusive result in a single trial
$(C_A - C_B) = 5\%$ with $C_B = 20\%$ & $C_A = 25\%$	$2N = 1\,000$	$2N = 1\,000$
$(C_A - C_B) = 10\%$ with $C_B = 40\%$ & $C_A = 50\%$	$2N = 400$	$2N = 700$
$(C_A - C_B) = 15\%$ with $C_B = 10\%$ & $C_A = 25\%$	$2N = 100$	$2N = 170$
$(C_A - C_B) = 20\%$ with $C_B = 20\%$ & $C_A = 40\%$	$2N = 75$	$2N = 130$

(Boag *et al., Brit J. Radiol.,* 1971, Vol. 44, p.122)

In a trial where a long term T-year survival rate, or a proportion cured, C, is the criterion, the analysis of results is undertaken after the 2N patients, Table 11.3, have entered the trial. The time lapse between the treatment of the final patient and the date of analysis will depend upon the method used to calculate the T-year rate, Chapter 10. In a *sequential trial*, however, the analysis continues throughout the duration of the trial, using a specially *designed chart* of which an example is given in Figure 11.2.

To describe the use of the chart in Figure 11.2, assume first that (*a*) the patient intake has been *paired*; (*b*) each member of the pair has been *randomised* into either a treatment A or treatment B group such that sometimes the first member of a pair will have A and sometimes the second member of a pair will have A; (*c*) a *criterion of success* has been defined and the treatment result of a pair is given one of the three ratings: (1) Treatment A better, (2) Treatment B better, (3) No difference.

Now consider the *first* patient pair. If A is better, a cross is made in the square immediately *above* the black square in the charts; but if B is better, a cross is made in the square immediately *to the right* of the black square; and if there is no difference, no entry is made in the charts. The results for the *second* and subsequent pairs are entered on the chart in a similar way using the square above or to the right of that marked for the preceding pair.

Once a *level of significance* has been chosen, such as $2\alpha = 0.20$ in Figure 11.2, this means an α-risk of 0.10 for A *better than* B and an α-risk of 0.10 for B *better than* A. It has already been stated that the *total patient intake* for the trial does not require prior specification and that a built-in *stopping rule* is a feature of any sequential analysis trial. The stopping rule is related to the *boundaries* of the square pattern of the Figure 11.2 chart, such that when the *upper boundary* is crossed the conclusion is that A is better than B, when the *lower boundary* is crossed, the conclusion is that B is better than A and when the *middle region* is entered, the conclusion is that *there is no difference between A and B*. This is illustrated in Figure 11.3.

Sequential trials are by no means limited to oncology and are particularly relevant when screening for drug specificity. However, before commencing such a trial, it is most important to ensure that the observations will be available for entering on the chart as soon as possible, since delay could mean extension beyond a stopping barrier and several patients unnecessarily receiving the poorer treatment. In this context it is essential not to make the matching characteristics for pairing too complicated, otherwise the trial will contain many unpaired patients and its duration may be unacceptably long.

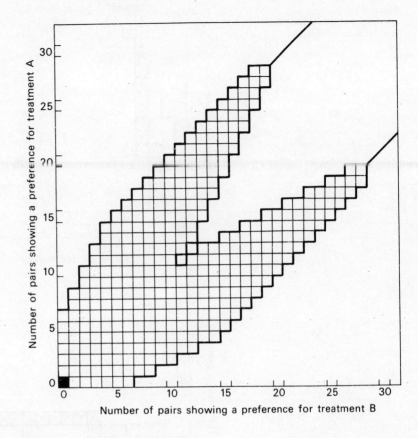

Figure 11.2
Sequential analysis chart with
an alpha risk of $2\alpha = 0.20$
*Courtesy: Ciba-Geigy Ltd.,
Basle, Switzerland.* See
also Bross, *Biometrics*,
1952, Vol. 8, 188—205.

Figure 11.3
Illustration of the stopping
rule for sequential trials

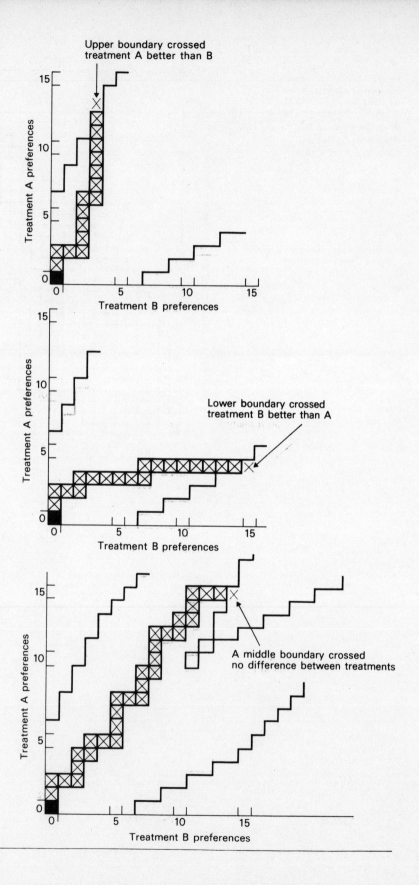

Glossary of Symbols

a	Slope (gradient) of a straight line, *see* Method of Least Squares, page 56.
b	Intercept of a straight line, *see* Method of Least Squares, page 56.
C	Proportion cured following treatment for cancer, pages 70 and 80. [C_A and C_B are the proportions cured for two different treatment groups A and B, page 83.]
^nC_r	Combinations of r from n. Symbol also denoted $\binom{n}{r}$, and it is also called the Binomial Coefficient, page 24
d_i, d_i^{CA}, d_i^{ID}	Numbers of deaths used in Life Table calculations, page 66. *see* also d_x, page 69.
E	Expected value, see chi-squared test where $\chi^2 = \dfrac{(O-E)^2}{E}$, page 40.

e Exponential symbol in a mathematical formula. e^x is called 'exponential to the power x' or 'e to the x' and is calculated from the series:

$$e^x = 1 + x + \frac{x^2}{2!} + \frac{x^3}{3!} + \dots\dots + \frac{x^N}{N!} \quad , (see \text{ Page } 11)$$

$\overset{o}{e}_x$	Life expectation, or average length of life, English Life Tables, page 69.
F	The F-statistic used in the F-test, page 51
H_o	The Null Hypothesis. [H_1 and H_2 are alternative hypotheses,] page 32.
l_i	Used in Life Table calculations, page 66. *See* also l_x, page 69.

$\text{Log}_e T$ 'Logarithm of T to base e'. Also called 'Natural Logarithms'. Logarithms may be calculated from the series:

$$\text{Log}_e(1+x) = x - \frac{x^2}{2} + \frac{x^3}{3} - \frac{x^4}{4} + \dots + (-1)^{N+1} \cdot \frac{x^N}{N}$$

and

$$\text{Log}_e(1-x) = -x - \frac{x^2}{2} - \frac{x^3}{3} - \frac{x^4}{4} - \dots - \frac{x^N}{N}$$

These formulae may only be used when x is in the range -1 to +1. Log Tables contain both Natural Logs. and Logs to Base 10.

$Log_{10}T$	'Logarithm of T to base 10'. (These are the *Logs* usually found in the first pages of school log tables). To convert from $Log_e T$ to $Log_{10}T$ use the formula:

$$Log_{10}T = \frac{Log_e T}{Log_e 10} \qquad \text{where } Log_e 10 = 2.3026$$

m_x	Death rate at age x, page 69
M	The parameter known as the mean of the Lognormal curve, page 12.
$N!$	'N factorial', calculated using the formula below:

$$
\begin{aligned}
1! &= 1 &&= 1 \\
2! &= 1 \times 2 &&= 2 \\
3! &= 1 \times 2 \times 3 &&= 6 \\
4! &= 1 \times 2 \times 3 \times 4 &&= 24
\end{aligned}
$$

$$\cdots\cdots\cdots$$

$$N! = 1 \times 2 \times 3 \times \ldots \times N$$

$n! \, (= 1 \times 2 \times 3 \times \ldots \times n)$ and $r! \, (= 1 \times 2 \times 3 \times \ldots \times r)$ are used in Chapter 5.

$N(t)$	Death rate of cases who die with cancer present, page 70.
n or N	Number of x-values, number of trials or experiments, ... etc.
n_i	Number of persons exposed to the risk of dying in the ith interval, used in Life Table calculations, page 66.
O	Observed value, see chi-squared test where $\chi^2 = \dfrac{(O\text{-}E)^2}{E}$
$_nP_r$	Permutations of r from n, page 23.
Pr	Probability. Pr [Success] is the 'probability of success of an experiment or trial', page 22.
P	Probability associated with the α-risk, e.g. $P=0.05$, $P=0.10$, page 35.
p	Binomial probability of success, page 24.
q	Binomial probability of failure, $(p+q) = 1$, page 24.
q_i	Probability of dying *in* the ith interval.
P_i	Probability of surviving *to* the end of the ith interval. q_i and P_i are used in Life Table calculations, page 66.
P_T	Probability of survival to time T, Life Table calculation, page 67.
p_x	Probability of living from age x to age $(x+1)$, English Life Tables, page 69.
q_x	Probability of dying in the year defined by the limits x and $(x+1)$, English Life Tables, page 69.

Q	Proportion of those cases who die with cancer present who die *after T* years have elapsed following treatment, page 70.
r	Correlation coefficient, page 59. It is also used in Chapter 5 when discussing Permutations and Combinations.
S_1, S_2	Standard deviations required for the F-test, page 51.
S	Standard deviation (this has been used in particular for the Lognormal curve, page 12), *see* also standard deviation of the difference in means, *t*-test, paired data, page 49.
t	The *t*-statistic used in the *t*-test, pages 48 and 59.
T	Survival time subsequent to treatment for cancer. *See* $\text{Log}_e T$ and the Lognormal curve. *T*-year survival rate, page 65.
w_i	Total cases lost to follow-up in the ith interval, used in Life Table calculations, page 66.
x	Age, English Life Tables, page 69, see also: l_x, d_x, p_x, q_x and $\overset{o}{e}_x$.
$(x_i, y_i), (X_i, Y_i)$	Co-ordinates of the ith point on a graph, pages 5 and 55.
$\bar{x}, \overline{X}$	Mean value of a series of *x*-values (or *X*-values)
x_i	The ith *x*-value in a series of *N* *x*-values: $x_1, x_2, \dots x_i, \dots x_N$.
$\bar{y}$	Mean value of a series of *y*-values.
Δy_i	Deviation of an observation (x_i, y_i) plotted as a point on a graph, from the best fit least squares straight line, page 58.
α	Alpha risk, page 34.
β	Beta risk, page 36. (1-β) is the Power of a test for significance, pages 81 and 82. β has also been used as a Binomial probability on page 42, [*see* also *p* and *q*].
Γ	A test statistic, page 38. (Gamma)
μ	The parameter known as the mean of the Normal curve, page 11. Also used as mean of the Binomial distribution, page 28, and as mean of the Poisson distribution, page 28. (Mu)
χ	Used in the chi-squared test as χ^2, page 40. (Chi)
π	A number equal to 3.1416. (Pi)
Σ	Sum of ..... (Sigma)
σ	Standard deviation (this has been used in particular for the Normal curve, page 11), see also standard deviation of the difference in means, *t*-test, unpaired data, page 50. (Sigma)
σ_a, σ_b	Standard errors in slope, *a*, and intercept, *b*, of a least squares best fit straight line, page 58.

ζ A particular value of X, when stating the area underneath a Normal curve between $X=-\infty$ and $X=\zeta$, see page 16. (Zeta)

ν Degrees of freedom for use with tests of significance, pages 41, 43, 47, 49, 50, 52, 59. (Nu)

∞ Infinity, page 16.

$\int$ An Integral sign. Mathematical notation in a formula when the area under a curve is being stated, page 15.

Books for Further Reading

Title	Author and Date of Publication	Publisher	Comments
1. *GENERAL STATISTICS*			
Statistical Methods in Medical Research	Armitage, P. (1973), 2nd Edn.	Blackwell, Oxford.	500 pages, 25 diagrams. At the same level as the present book.
Principles of Medical Statistics	Hill, A. Bradford (1971), 9th Edn.	*The Lancet,* London	400 pages, 20 diagrams. 1st Edn. published 1937. Extends into greater detail than the present book.
Statistics in Small Doses	Castle, W.M., (1972)	Churchill Livingstone, Edinburgh	225 pages, 170 diagrams. At same level as the present book, written completely in a *question and answer format.*
2. *STATISTICAL TABLES*			
Statistical Tables for Biological, Agricultural and Medical Research	Fisher, R.A. and Yates, F. (1974), 6th Edn.	Longman, London.	*Standard reference book* of statistical tables, 146 pages.
Cambridge Elementary Statistical Tables	Lindley, D.V. and Miller J.C.P. (1968)	Cambridge University Press.	35 pages only, but all the most useful tables in adequate detail. *Inexpensive.*
3. *STATISTICS WITH EXAMPLES DRAWN MAINLY FROM A SPECIFIC FIELD*			
Basic statistics in *Behavioural Research*	Maxwell, A.E. (1972)	Penguin	120 pages, 10 diagrams. Contains no data on clinical trails.
Experiment, design and statistics in *Psychology*	Robsón, C. (1973)	Penguin	175 pages, 20 diagrams. Contains *step-by-step* worked examples.
Statistics for *Biology*	Bishop, O. (1971)	Longman, London.	220 pages, 20 diagrams.
Primer of *Epidemiology*	Friedman, G.D. (1974)	McGraw-Hill, New York.	230 pages, 25 diagrams. Minimal basic statistical theory.

Title	Author and Date of Publication	Publisher	Comments
Medical Research, a statistical and *epidemiological* approach	England, J.M. (1975)	Churchill Livingstone, Edinburgh.	200 pages, 80 diagrams. Less introductory statistics than the present book.
Mathematics and statistics for use in the *biological and pharmaceutical industries*	Saunders, L. and Fleming, R. (1971)	The Pharmaceutical Press, London	310 pages, 45 diagrams. At a higher level than the present book.

4. *CLINICAL TRIALS*

Sequential Medical Trials	Armitage, P. (1975), 2nd Edn.	Blackwell, Oxford.	200 pages, 20 diagrams. Specialised book.
The Principles and Practice of Clinical Trials	Harris, E.L. and Fitzgerald, J.D. (Editors), (1970)	Livingstone, Edinburgh.	250 pages, 75 diagrams. Conference proceedings. Specialised book.

Author Index

Subject Index

incidence, 76
prevalence, 76
survival, 76
Tests
    chi-squared, 40
    critical value of test statistic, 38
    degrees of freedom, 38, 41, 43, 47, 49, 50, 52
    difference in means, 48
    difference in proportions, 44
    difference in standard deviations, 51
    difference in variances, 51
    F-test, 51
    one-tailed and two-tailed, 35, 61
    parametric and non-parametric, 48
    power of a test, 81
    robust, 48, 51
    significant correlation, 59
    t-test, 48, 59
    test statistic, 38
Theorem, central limit, 38
Traffic accidents, 63
Transformation, 13
Trend, 53
Trial
    alpha and beta risks, *see* Alpha risk and
       Beta risk
    bias, 79
    binomial conditions, 25
    blind, 78
    clinical trial, 78
    decision making, 78
    null hypothesis, 31, Fig. 6.1, 34, 37, 41, 43
    number of patients required in a trial, 80, 81
    paired, 27, 81, Fig. 11.2, Fig. 11.3
    power of a test, 81, 82
    proportion cured, 70, Fig. 10.1, 73, 81
    randomisation, 79
    sequential analysis, 83
Tuberculosis, 62
Two-tailed test, 35, 61
Type I error, 33
Type II error, 33
Typhoid innoculation, 46

U

Unpaired *t*-test, 50

V

Variance, 9, Fig. 2.2

W

Weight gain, 50
Worked examples
    binomial probabilities, 26, 27, 42
    chi-squared (χ^2) test, curve fitting, 44
    chi-squared test, frequency table, 40
    combinations, 24
    2 x 2 contingency table (χ^2), 45-47
    correlation coefficient, 60
    correlation coefficient and *t*-test, 61
    cumulative frequency, 3
    direct method of calculating survival rates, 67
    F-test, 51
    laws of mathematical probability, 20, 21, 22
    least squares method, slope and intercept, 57
    Life Table method of calculating survival
      rates, 65-68
    Mean, 7
    Mean, Mode and Median for slightly asym-
      metric curves, 8
    Mean and standard deviation using arithmetic
      probability graph paper for the normal
      curve and logarithmic probability graph
      paper for the lognormal curve, 18
    Median, 8
    Mode 7
    paired *t*-test, 49
    Pascal's triangle, 26
    percentage cumulative frequency, 3
    permutations, 23
    Poisson probabilities, 29
    probability of success of an operation, 22
    probability and area under the normal
      curve, 21
    significance tables, how to read them, 38
    standard deviation (two methods), 10
    standard deviation and probability, 16
    standard deviation and area under a normal
      curve, 16
    straight line slope and intercept, 57
    survival rate calculation, direct method, 67
    survival rate calculation, life table method,
      65-68
    time in equal logarithmic intervals to base
      1.5, 13
    unpaired *t*-test, 50